A Tale of a Man, a \
a Snail

The Schistosomiasis Control Initiative

A TALE OF A MAN, A WORM AND A SNAIL

The Schistosomiasis Control Initiative

by

Alan Fenwick
Imperial College London, UK

Wendie Norris
Formerly CABI, UK

Becky McCall
Freelance medical journalist, UK

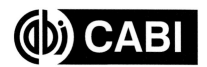

CABI is a trading name of CAB International

CABI
Nosworthy Way
Wallingford
Oxfordshire OX10 8DE
UK

Tel: +44 (0)1491 832111
Fax: +44 (0)1491 833508
E-mail: info@cabi.org
Website: www.cabi.org

CABI
WeWork
One Lincoln St
24th Floor
Boston, MA 02111
USA

T: +1 (617)682-9015
E-mail: cabi-nao@cabi.org

A catalogue record for this book is available from the British Library, London, UK.

Library of Congress Cataloging-in-Publication Data

Names: Fenwick, Alan, author.
Title: A tale of a man, a worm and a snail : the schistosomiasis control
    initiative / Alan Fenwick, Wendie Norris, Becky McCall.
Description: Wallingford, Oxfordshire ; Boston, MA : CAB International,
    [2022] | Includes bibliographical references and index. | Summary:
    "Schistosomiasis is Africa's second most prevalent infectious disease
    after malaria and is a neglected tropical disease. This book offers a
    unique perspective on a successful health initiative that can serve as a
    model for other diseases. It will be of interest to those working in
    global health and disease control"-- Provided by publisher.
Identifiers: LCCN 2021033331 (print) | LCCN 2021033332 (ebook) | ISBN
    9781786392558 (pap erback) | ISBN 9781786392565 (ebook) | ISBN
    9781786392572 (epub)
Subjects: LCSH: Schistosomiasis. | Medicine, Preventive.
Classification: LCC RA644.S3 F46 2022 (print) | LCC RA644.S3 (ebook) |
    DDC 614.5/53--dc23
LC record available at https://lccn.loc.gov/2021033331
LC ebook record available at https://lccn.loc.gov/2021033332

References to Internet websites (URLs) were accurate at the time of writing.

ISBN-13: 9781786392558 (paperback)
          9781786392565 (ePDF)
          9781786392572 (ePub)

DOI: 10.1079/9781786392558.0000

Commissioning Editor: Alexandra Lainsbury
Editorial Assistant: Lauren Davies
Production Editor: Marta Patiño

Typeset by Exeter Premedia Services Pvt Ltd. Chennai, India
Printed and bound in the UK by Severn, Gloucester

Contents

I would like to dedicate this book to my closest family. To my wife Margie. To my three daughters Janet, Gill, and Helen, and my sister Marney.

Foreword

Peter Hotez

Across the globe, the name Alan Fenwick and the disease that comprises his life's work, schistosomiasis, are not yet household words. They probably should be. Perhaps no other person has been so singularly connected to the control of schistosomiasis over these last 60 years, while there is now abundant evidence that schistosomiasis represents a global health threat equivalent to malaria, HIV/AIDS, or even COVID-19.

Since the early 1960s, when Alan first travelled to Africa, he has been at the forefront of global schistosomiasis control. Today, schistosomiasis remains one of the most common and devastating afflictions of humankind. The actual number of people who harbour adult schistosome worms in their blood vessels or schistosome eggs (each armed with a spine) in their tissues is not fully known. This is partly because the disease is mostly found in rural villages across the African continent, but estimates range from 200 million to possibly 400 million forgotten people.

Here are some examples of the human destruction: schistosome eggs damage the cervix, uterus and lower genital tract of millions of adolescent girls and young women, causing daily misery due to bleeding, pain, social stigma and depression. The condition now known as female genital schistosomiasis is a leading gynaecological condition in Africa, which has been identified as a major co-factor in Africa's HIV/AIDS epidemic. Those eggs also cause damage to the bladder resulting in bleeding such that on any given day tens of millions of children and adolescents pass blood in their urine. In the longer term, schistosomes cause serious pathology of the bladder, leading to cancer; and to the intestines and liver, causing high blood pressure; and is a major reason why children cannot grow to their full intellectual and physical potential.

Alan's first job in 1966 was in Tanzania, but he continued in Africa for more than five decades, living in Sudan and Egypt, and then working in Mali, Niger, Burkina Faso, Uganda and Zambia. Alan saw first-hand how schistosomiasis destroyed a generation of African men and women. He ultimately had a leading role in just about every approach to the control of this disease, including snail control, vaccine development, behavioural change and mass drug administration with praziquantel. Reading *A Tale of a Man, a Worm and a Snail: The Schistosomiasis Control Initiative* is a ticket to a front seat for every international effort attempted over the last six decades to reduce the public health impact of this disease in Africa. It culminates in the fascinating story of how Alan used his expertise, his credibility, his track record of success and finally his extraordinary force of personality to persuade a newly created Bill & Melinda Gates Foundation to make a major investment in praziquantel mass drug administration and provide the essential seed funding to create the Schistosomiasis Control Initiative (SCI).

Today, SCI is one of the premier non-governmental development organizations devoted to neglected tropical diseases, with an unparalleled almost 20 years of successes in reducing the disease burden of schistosomiasis. Under Alan's able leadership, and now through his long-time associate and successor, Dr Wendy Harrison, hundreds of millions of people annually receive access to essential medicines for schistosomiasis and related parasitic infections. SCI works across Africa to provide these treatments and desperately needed technical assistance to health ministries. In so doing, SCI has become an international treasure and one of our most vital and important global health organizations.

I joined Professor Fenwick on his journey and quest in 2003, just following the inception of SCI. It has been a true privilege for me to work with Alan and learn from him these past two decades as we joined forces with our mutual friend and colleague, Professor David Molyneux. Our group of global health 'three musketeers' helped to create a neglected tropical diseases (NTDs) framework linking treatments for the high-prevalence parasitic and related infections. Now SCI and other UK-based organizations, including Sightsavers, Uniting to Combat NTDs, The Liverpool School of Tropical Medicine, and DFID and UK AID, are at the forefront of NTD control, advocacy and training. They all collaborate together with a group of leading organizations on the North American side of the Atlantic Ocean, including the Task Force for Global Health, RTI, FHI 360, The End Fund, USAID, and others. As a result, in collaboration with the World Health Organization, now more than one billion people receive annual access to essential medicines for NTDs.

One of my favourite parts of Alan's life story is his boyhood, growing up in Liverpool with a friendship group including John Lennon, and being there when Lennon and Paul McCartney first met. My guided tour of the Beatles' Liverpool and spending time with Alan and his wife Margaret Wright on many occasions are among my favourite memories. Alan Fenwick may not be quite as celebrated as the Beatles, but his contributions to the health of African people living in extreme poverty have left an indelible mark. He is in every way a hero for his contributions to lift the poorest people out of poverty through science and medicine.

Peter Hotez, MD, PhD, Professor and Dean,
National School of Tropical Medicine,
Baylor College of Medicine, Houston, Texas

Foreword: Changing People's Lives

The Schistosomiasis Control Initiative was established in 2002 and was hosted by Imperial College London for 17 years. During that time, SCI established schistosomiasis and intestinal worm treatment programmes in 16 countries and assisted those countries to deliver over 200 million treatments, mainly through schools, to cleanse the human population of worms.

To illustrate the effect that SCI had in these countries and on the staff involved, I have invited four individuals to tell us what SCI meant to them and to the health of their country's population.

Dr Seydou Touré, Dr Narcis Kabatereine and Dr Amadou Garba were, in 2002, junior staff members of the ministries of health in Burkina Faso, Uganda and Niger, respectively. They had a minimal working budget, no access to medicines and no vehicles, yet they were each their own country's bilharzia control officer (bilharzia is an alternative name for schistosomiasis).

SCI went to each country, worked with them, and 17 years later they had overseen the treatment of all school-age children and have risen from their junior status to being very successful in their careers.

Dr Albis Gabrielli joined SCI early in his career as a francophone programme manager and later joined WHO in the Neglected Tropical Diseases control unit.

Each has told their story in the form of a letter to show what SCI has meant to them.

Alan Fenwick

Burkina Faso

In 2002 I had no idea what an effect the visit of the SCI team to Ouagadougou would have on the health of the population of Burkina Faso and on my career. At that time I was a junior member of the staff of the Ministry of Health, with responsibility for the control of bilharzia. SCI had written to say they wanted to help some countries in Africa to treat their infected populations with praziquantel. I knew about this drug but we had no funds in our budget to buy it. I was aware of the high prevalence of bilharzia in Burkina Faso and the extent of blood in the urine of schoolchildren so I invited SCI to visit. When I asked my minister of health to meet them he was a bit sceptical. In the past, teams had visited the ministry but expected us to host them in hotels and meet their expenses, and after they left we reaped no benefit from their visit. Professor Fenwick and Mr Howard Thompson were very different. They met all their own expenses and explained their plan to HE Alain Yoda, our Minister – SCI wanted Burkina to be an example country in which the ministry team would arrange to map infections, provide health education and plan treatments in all infected areas. SCI would provide funds for these interventions and provide the praziquantel for bilharzia and albendazole to deworm our children. Frankly, we could not believe it, but we decided to give SCI a chance. Thank God we did! Over the next six years all the children in Burkina Faso were treated by the ministry (with the help of the French NGO RISEAL) and the improvement in health was measured. My minister was so thrilled that he arranged, in 2006, for Professor Fenwick, Mr Thompson and the SCI staff member Dr Gabrielli to receive a medal from our country. He included Dr Bertrand Sellin from RISEAL. As for me, I was also thrilled with SCI for giving me the resources to arrange all the treatments and to work with my counterparts from Niger and Mali. For a relatively small investment in my country SCI improved the health of millions of people – and my reputation in my ministry.

Seydou Touré, MD, MPH,
Chevalier de l'Ordre National

Working on the Inside – for SCI

I joined the Schistosomiasis Control Initiative during the summer of 2003. I remember that I found the vacancy notice on Imperial College's website just a couple of days after the deadline had passed. I wrote to the generic e-mail address shown on the website and asked if I could still apply. After a few hours, Alan (who I didn't know then) replied affirmatively. That was the beginning of the adventure. A few days later I flew to London for the interview and that's when I met Alan, together with Howard Thompson, Joanne Webster and Kieran Bird. SCI was very young and small then; Lynsey Blair and Christine Selfe completed the team. A few weeks later I was offered the job and moved to London.

My title was Programme Manager for West Africa and I was following up on SCI's activities in three countries: Burkina Faso, Mali and Niger. Lynsey was in charge of three additional countries in eastern and southern Africa: Uganda, Tanzania and Zambia.

A few weeks later came my first travel to West Africa, with Howard, and Bertrand and Elisabeth Sellin, two French scientists with a long-standing experience of schistosomiasis in Africa. We met with officials in the three countries and started making arrangements for SCI's operations, including recruiting local staff, identifying an office and buying a car. I was young and everything looked immensely interesting to me.

Things started to move quickly and in early 2004 we had completed purchase of praziquantel (no donation programmes back then) and established excellent relations with the health authorities in the three countries. Activities were launched through high-level, colourful events, after which treatment successfully started and rapidly scaled up. We were making a difference.

If I think about those days now, I am surprised how things seemed to proceed smoothly, and how quickly ideas were followed by action. I believe that our strength was the excellent teamwork between SCI and the national counterparts, and also the strong balance between science and operations, deskwork and fieldwork.

We had three excellent programme managers in charge of schistosomiasis within the ministries of health in each of the countries: Seydou Touré in Burkina Faso, Robert Dembélé in Mali and Amadou Garba in Niger. They could rely on high-level support within their respective governments as well as on many others joining forces and contributing: Moussa Sacko, Aly Landouré, Jean-Noël Poda, Césaire Ky, Malachie Yaogho, Adama Keita, among others.

Back in London, Alan was overseeing everything with his characteristic style, demanding but light-hearted, sensible and wise, full of commonsense and understanding of everyone. I enjoyed working with him, because even though he was tough and direct sometimes, there was always a good purpose behind the toughness. I knew that he was doing it to improve my capacities and enable me to grow up.

Behind Alan's strong leadership we had an equally strong team that included, in addition to those mentioned above, Russell Stothard, Archie Clements, Sarah Whawell, Cara Kamenka, Artemis Koukounari and, later on, Elisa Bosqué-Oliva, Yaobi Zhang, Fiona Fleming, James Hammersley, and others.

As for me, the two years I spent at SCI were among the best of my life, both from a human and a professional perspective, and what I learned then has remained as a lasting and ever-renewed legacy.

Albis Gabrielli
Regional Adviser,
Neglected Tropical Diseases,
WHO Egypt

Uganda

My Dream

Alan, you have indeed changed the lives of numerous people, including mine.

I completed my BSc degree in Makerere University, Uganda, in 1978 and joined the Ministry of Health, Vector Control Division, in 1980. The division houses the NTD programme. I was told to work on bilharzia (schistosomiasis), and I got confused. Was there bilharzia in Uganda? At the university we had studied bilharzia but as a disease of Gezira (Sudan) and Egypt. No one talked of bilharzia in Uganda. Next, I was given files to read as I prepared to embark on the work. I read publications by George Nelson, David Bradley, V.L. Ongom and M. Prentice, all showing that schistosomiasis was a severe problem in Uganda, but neglected. No one was working on it. Prentice, a British citizen in whose former office I now sat, had started on it and had written in one paper that 'Uganda was a cradle of schistosomes'. Professor Ongom had published thrilling manuscripts on schistosomiasis morbidity in Uganda but died before doing anything to control it. I am told his death was related to bilharzia late complications. There was no one to consult, and instead I had to take the bull by its horns, alone. I attended a bilharzia course at Danish Bilharziasis Laboratory in Denmark in 1983.

Equipped with the necessary knowledge, I was eager to embark on the long journey of bilharzia control in Uganda, but I had no funds. I embarked on fundraising, mainly from local NGOs and sometimes I would get a little money. I used every cent to map out snail vectors and collect data on the epidemiology of the disease. By 2000, I had much data and had also acquired a PhD in the epidemiology of schistosomiasis, but I still had no funds to control the disease, even in a single village.

The Disease in Uganda

Schistosomiasis mansoni had been known for a long time along the shores of Lake Albert and the Albert Nile in north-western Uganda. It was first detected at the beginning of the last century; cases were reported from 1923, but thorough studies only occurred between 1950 and 1959, in the early 1970s, and mine in the 1990s. All these studies showed that the disease was a serious problem and widespread, particularly within the Albert/Nile basin. One of the studies described the disease to be very intense, more so than any other area ever studied. Hospital records over a 30-year period between 1951 and 1980 showed this condition to be the first cause of hospital death and the second cause of hospital admissions in adults.

However, until after SCI support, knowledge about the disease among over 99% of health specialists was as poor as in the communities they served. Schistosomiasis management was left to traditional healers with payments in the form of goats, chicken and money from victims, even though they had no cure. Their patients would end up in hospitals to die, since our health system could not manage severe disease. Traditional healers did not know the cause of the disease they claimed to cure. Ascites was commonly attributed to witchcraft and the reported witches were usually old women or widows without defence, and most ended up being killed by mobs in revenge for many deaths that were caused. Many people vomited blood (haematemesis) before death and traditional healers claimed it was punishment from the gods for stealing people's fishnets. Schistosomiasis control relies on a thorough understanding of the epidemiology of the disease, but there were no funds for research. The situation was similar elsewhere in sub-Saharan Africa. I met Alan Fenwick in 2002, after almost two decades of such frustrations.

My First Meeting with Alan Fenwick

We were in Zambia attending a WHO AFRO Workshop on bilharzia control facilitated by the late Dr Likezo Mubila, a long-time friend. I got to know Alan from someone who shouted his name in excitation on seeing him. I had read and admired his work in Tanzania, Sudan and Egypt. I made it my goal to meet him to persuade him to work in Uganda too. I got my chance to talk to him after dinner when he was alone taking coffee. I asked if he was the Fenwick I had read about in Sudan and Egypt and he answered in the affirmative. In our talk, I realized he needed a country with data on schistosomiasis where he could work, while I had data and desperately needed financial support. We became friends, and after the workshop he accompanied me to Uganda to attend a World Food Programme workshop in Entebbe, where I was expected to present my data to justify the need for deworming in WFP food-supported schools. We discussed my data and Alan took a copy, promising support if he got funds.

SCI Support to Uganda in Schistosomiasis and Worm Control

His proposal got funded by the Bill & Melinda Gates Foundation, and towards the end of 2002, I learnt that Uganda would be among the first countries to benefit. He had formed an NGO, Schistosomiasis Control Initiative, attached to Imperial College London, and the support was to reach us through that NGO. In 2003, our first Schistosomiasis and Worm Control Programme was launched by the deputy prime minister of Uganda, Moses Ali, accompanied by 40 members of parliament, the minister of health, several dignitaries from WHO and other stakeholders. By 2004 we had mapped the distribution and magnitude of schistosomiasis in the country. By 2006, all foci with a prevalence above 20% were receiving annual MDAs. Currently, Uganda is among group 1 countries whose goal is interruption of transmission in foci where transmission occurs on small water bodies. Here morbidity has been eliminated. Over 140 publications have been produced, mainly on the epidemiology of the disease. Between 2011 and 2018 I was employed by SCI as African Capacity Building Advisor and I travelled widely and frequently, attending most of the important meetings on schistosomiasis. I have carried out a large number of WHO consultancies at regional and headquarters level, I have participated in a number of WHO working groups and am a member of NTD RPRG for NTD control at WHO/AFRO Region. Currently, I am employed by ASCEND (Accelerating the Sustainable Control and Elimination of Neglected Tropical Diseases) as Country Lead, Uganda. All these achievements are attributed to Alan Fenwick's support, for which I will be forever grateful.

Narcis Bujune Kabatereine
ASCEND Country Lead, Uganda

Niger

My first meeting with Alan was during a training workshop organized by WHO in Niamey in January 2001. The reason why Niamey was chosen was the long experience of the research centre there, named CERMES – the specialized centre in schistosomiasis research of OCCGE (organisation de coordination et de coopération pour la lutte contre les grandes endémies), a West African research centre network. I was a trainer at the workshop, and I was in charge of organizing the fieldwork for the participants. The field experience given by me made Alan realize the highest prevalence of the disease in this sub-region, but also to discover the existing francophone expertise in schistosomiasis. I think this, among other reasons, explains the decision to include Mali, Niger and Burkina Faso among the countries to be supported by the newly created Schistosomiasis Control Initiative.

Before SCI, lots of experts were doubtful of the impact of mass drug administration strategy to control and eliminate schistosomiasis as a public health problem because of the cost of praziquantel (the drug used to treat schistosomiasis) and also because of re-infection of the treated people after treatment: therefore, many governments did not want to invest in a programme requiring long-term support. Alan and SCI showed that it is possible to have great impact on the morbidity of the disease through treatment with praziquantel and, moreover, showed that it is possible to scale up schistosomiasis control activities, countrywide, to all people in need, at a reasonable cost.

The SCI programme allowed Niger, Mali and Burkina to establish a control programme and to provide treatment to tens of millions of school-age children, but also to adults whose occupations put them at risk of schistosomiasis (rice growers, fishermen, women etc.), and avoid the disease progressing towards complications and death.

Moreover, SCI expanded the support to establish, for the first time, integrated neglected tropical disease programmes targeting, in addition to schistosomiasis, other diseases such as lymphatic filariasis, trachoma, onchocerciasis and soil-transmitted helminths for more efficiency of the medicine distribution campaign. It is important to highlight that Alan and SCI also offered the opportunity to these countries (Mali, Niger and Burkina) to strengthen their collaborations with disease-control local expertise (through RISEAL).

The tremendous contribution of Alan to public health was recognized by the governments of Burkina Faso and Niger through the award of high distinction medals to him and his team.

The support of Alan in the creation of the national schistosomiasis control programme in Niger was the opportunity for me to move from research to programme implementation as co-ordinator of the schistosomiasis programme. It offers me opportunities to meet with other researchers and set collaborations beyond the francophone world. Those early SCI years have been a very productive period, with many publications on schistosomiasis, with Alan's support to operational research studies. This research contributed to the improvement of the WHO strategies for control of the morbidity, monitoring, evaluation and management of schistosomiasis programmes.

Amadou Garba
RISEAL Niger,
Réseau International
Schistosomiases Environnement

Preface

For the uninitiated, schistosomiasis, also known as bilharzia, is a disease caused by a parasitic worm which invades the human body when aquatic snails, which are the intermediate host of the worms, release larvae into the water. These larvae can penetrate the unbroken skin of people who are in contact with that water. The larvae become adult worms in the liver, which pair up (male and female) and then migrate to live in blood vessels around the bladder or intestine. Their lifespan can be 5–30 years. It is a horribly widespread, debilitating disease causing untold suffering to the victim and, ultimately, if untreated, death.

The Purpose of this Book

During my working life, which, in the main, has been dedicated to fighting this disease, I have had the good fortune of meeting some wonderful people, enjoying some great adventures and lighter moments. This book is the story of my life but it also concentrates on the achievements of the single initiative I founded, the Schistosomiasis Control Initiative (SCI). Along the way I hope to introduce you to a selection of those people and share some of those adventures and anecdotes as we focused on a common cause. That's the success story I want to tell – but let's start with the parasite that never ceases to amaze me, the schistosome worm, and the just-as-amazing continent of Africa and its people with whom I have spent such a wonderful career.

The first 26 years of my life was spent in the UK, the next five years in Tanzania, followed by 17 years in Sudan and then 14 years in Egypt. Then, in 2002, I returned to the UK and joined Imperial College London as Professor of Tropical Parasitology and Founder and Director of the SCI. In 2017 I retired from SCI and handed over control and in 2019 I retired from Imperial College as an Emeritus Professor.

In telling my story I hope to relate to the reader the many learnings and achievements of my period overseas culminating in the establishment of SCI, a major initiative with funding initially provided by the Bill and Melinda Gates Foundation (Gates Foundation). SCI, based at and hosted by Imperial College from 2002 to 2019, provides a success story of expansion and collaboration which has resulted in almost every country in Africa trying to first control schistosomiasis and intestinal worms as public health problems and then proceed to their elimination.

Acknowledgements

I owe so much to so many people who have supported and encouraged me during my life and without whom I would not have a story to tell. On a personal level, my heartfelt gratitude is to my wife and partner Margie, who has been by my side with patience and inspiration throughout my directorship of SCI and writing this book. My warmest appreciation goes to Irene, mother of our three daughters Janet, Gill and Helen, for her support in my early working years in Tanzania and Sudan.

Over the years, and in many countries, I have collaborated with inspirational people, especially David Molyneux and Peter Hotez, and gathered many wonderful friends who have filled my life with richness and stories. To them I am very thankful.

This book started life as a scientific textbook in 2007 with the help of my ghostwriter Becky McCall, but we did not finish it, and the almost-completed manuscript lay dormant for several years during the busy expansion time with SCI. I am very grateful to Penny Perrins at CABI who, together with Alex Lainsbury, pushed me to complete the book they had agreed to publish. I decided to finalize the manuscript after I retired from SCI in 2018, but was encouraged by my successor at SCI, Dr Wendy Harrison, to include some anecdotes about the development of SCI and its success story. As the book developed, I sent drafts to Di Donaldson, a great friend and avid reader, who lives in Cape Town, and who urged me to finish the book and made some excellent editorial comments. The same is true of Dr Joe Cook in the USA who read an early draft.

CABI very kindly assigned a professional editor, Wendie Norris, their own Global Health Specialist, to take the book to publication, and her intervention turned this book around with her incredibly professional input. I had no idea how much extra work this would involve, but five or six versions later we are there. Thank you Wendie and all who have contributed to the writing, editing and publishing of this book.

Thanks are also due to Dr Amadou Garba for providing maps and data.

I would like to express my thanks to the thousands of people who have donated to SCI over the last 17 years. Some large donors like the Bill and Melinda Gates Foundation, and Luke Ding, Legatum and the End Fund, but also many individuals who donated to SCI. More recently, Luke Ding, Legatum and Merck, through the Global Schistosomiasis Alliance, have offered funding towards the publication of this book. You have all made such a difference to the health of children in Africa.

The work of SCI was to help the ministries of health and education in 16 countries to treat their infected and at-risk populations, and so our gratitude and special mention must go to all the local people of the countries in Africa who have put their faith and trust in SCI. To the ministers of health and education, to their schistosomiasis control teams and to the schoolteachers in all the schools, a huge vote of thanks for their efforts.

And to the 200 million recipients of praziquantel and albendazole, my thanks for trusting us and coming forward for treatment. Without them, the ministries, control teams and teachers, and without the contribution of an excellent and dynamic team of people, SCI would not exist. Below I have named, in alphabetical order by first name, all those who have worked at SCI at Imperial College.

Albis Gabrielli, Alice Norton, Alix Grainger, Amadou Garba, Anna Phillips, Anna Wilhelme, Annalan Navaratnam, Anouk Gouvras, Antonio Zivieri, Archie Clements, Arminder Deol, Beatriz Calvo, Ben Styles, Blandine Labry, Bozena Marchelewicz, Bradley Gant, Cara Kamenka, Carlos Torres, Carolyn Henry, Christine Logan, Christine Selfe, Claire Wright, Claudia Pisani, Cristina Young, Demran Ali, Dhekra Annazaili, Elana Andreisheva, Fiona Fleming, Giuseppina Ortu, Howard Thompson, Jacqui Leslie, Jane Whitton, Jaya Shrivastava, Jemima Hills, Joanne Webster, Katie Fantaguzzi, Kieran Bird, Lazanya Weekes, Lei Zhang, Lindsey Cole, Liz Hollenberg, Lotte Gower, Lynsey Blair, Marie-Aimee Sandrine, Marie-Alice Deville, Marisol Granados, Michael French, Michelle Clements, Mike Hauser, Mousoumi Rahman, Moussa Sacko, Nadia Ben Meriem, Nadine Seward, Najwa Al Abdallah, Narcis Kabatereine, Neerav Dhahani, Nick Baldry, Pedro Gazzinelli, Peter Dranfield, Peter Jourdan, Peter Nelson, Poppy Lamberton, Roya Karimnia, Russell Stothard, Sam Zaramba, Sarah Knowles, Sarah Nogaro, Sarah Whawell, Scott Gordon, Seydou Touré, Shaivali Shah, Udo Wittmann, Wendy Harrison, Yael Velleman, Yaobi Zhang, Yolissa Nalule.

I hope that you will get to read the book and recognize the contribution you have all made to the success of SCI and the improvement of the health of millions of children in Africa.

Prologue: An Elephant Study by a Lake Sets Me on a New Path

It was yet another beautiful African day in Arusha, Tanzania, as I stood by the side of a pool at the campsite of Ian Douglas Hamilton collecting snails on the edge of Lake Manyara National Park. The pool was located at the foot of a waterfall rushing water down the Manyara escarpment, and the overflow from this pool then flowed down as the Ndala river to Lake Manyara.

Ian had contracted bilharzia, something that I was studying as Research Officer for the TPRI. He had been passing unusually huge numbers of parasite eggs in his stool, and his physician, Dr David Brooke, had called me in (as the local expert) to investigate. I was intrigued enough to follow up the case to find out how and where he had contracted this most terrible of diseases.

I asked him about where he was living, where he worked and what water contact he might have, i.e. his lifestyle and any exposure to fresh water. It turned out he had built a camp in the National Park, with the permission of the Head of National Parks John Owen, to enable him to study for his PhD at Oxford University, and for this study he was painstakingly photographing every elephant in the park and identifying them from the shapes of their ears.

Once Ian had recovered from the treatment, I went back with him to his house in the park to try to work out how he had managed to acquire such a heavy infection, but I needed to know if this was an exclusive event or if it went broader and touched others in the area.

It was not too difficult, because he had sited his house on the banks of a small river, so I immediately collected snails from the pool right next to his house.

I could not believe how many hundreds of *Biomphalaria pfeifferi* snails I collected from that pool, nor how many of them were shedding cercariae, the free-swimming larvae which infect humans in contact with the water.

Ian said that he and his guests, when he had some, all bathed in this pool every morning, which I could see would be a recipe for a massive infection with bilharzia. Over the next few days I took in the situation, and during one night I heard a troop of baboons turn up and roost above the pool in the overhanging trees.

The next morning their faeces were all around and so I collected some samples of these, too, and examined them microscopically. They were all full of *S. mansoni* eggs. Despite not realizing the importance of this finding, I was incredibly excited about the situation; I wondered where this massive contamination could have come from, and who other than Ian might have been unknowingly infected.

Fortunately, Ian had kept a visitors book, and he allowed me to contact all the people who had stayed at his camp, some for just one night and some for longer. By mail, I asked them whether they had suffered diarrhoea around 5–8 weeks after their visit to Lake Manyara. I also realized that the more recent visitors might be infected but that the worms would not yet be laying eggs, so I warned them of the possibility of future symptoms. As it happened, two of the recent visitors were John Owen's two young children who had stayed with Ian for several nights during their Easter vacation from their UK boarding school. I suspected they would be very heavily infected and could become very seriously ill. I calculated when the infection would mature (into worms laying eggs) and wrote to their school in the UK. It was a good job we took this precaution because 40 days after their stay in Manyara they developed massive diarrhoea and bloody stools. With the diagnosis made in advance, the school was ready, and the two girls (aged 12 and 10) were treated quickly and recovered well. That might not have been the case without the warning because doctors in the UK might never have thought of bilharzia as a cause of their symptoms.

Every one of the other guests who had stayed in the camp responded to my enquiry, and it turned out that anyone who had bathed after 1 April had suffered the same symptoms, while those who bathed earlier than that date did not get infected. Knowing that infection in the snail matures about six weeks after infection, I asked Ian what had happened at the camp in mid-February. It turned out that a group of local men camped there for several days while thatching the roof of Ian's new house, and I concluded that they had used the pool for their ablutions and had probably introduced the infection into the pool and infected the snails for the first time. The first infection in the snails had matured on 1 April, and from then on the pond was incredibly heavily infected. The baboons had become infected while drinking and even eating snails, and maintained the cycle of infection, and so Ian and his guests became the main human sufferers.

I asked John Owen for, and was granted, approval for a special scientific study to complete the proof of baboons being infected. This permitted one of their rangers to shoot six baboons from the troop and for a vet to be with me to carry out a *post mortem* to prove whether they were harbouring worms and that the eggs were viable. On successive days we were able to shoot three baboons and on *post mortem* all three were infected with schistosomes identical to *S. mansoni*.

Those animals were smart and they soon learnt that we were dangerous. From day 4 onwards they scattered whenever they heard a vehicle approach and we failed to get a shot at another animal. I really felt that I needed the six to provide the necessary conclusive evidence, so we persevered and decided to try trapping the remaining three overnight in cages. Our cage, with a banana as bait, was effective on day 1 and we examined our fourth baboon, which proved to be infected also. But the next morning, instead of another baboon, we found that the cage had disappeared because the animals had picked it up and thrown it into the river! (I did say they were smart). So we staked the next cage securely and managed baboon number 5. From then on the bait disappeared every night but without a baboon getting caught.

Finally, we did trap baboon number 6, but as this turned out to be a pregnant female, we released her. It was a good job we did, because literally 15 minutes after her release, a Land Rover pulled up at the camp carrying two people who were visiting Ian; it was Bill Travers and Virginia McKenna, the two wildlife-loving film stars. So we quickly settled for five baboons, 100% infected, and I was able to tell the story and publish the demonstration that baboons under special circumstances could maintain transmission of bilharzia in nature. This story turned out to be quite unique and so the study was published as a scientific paper and formed a chapter of my PhD thesis a couple of years later.

The study was to have long-term and life-changing consequences for me and my life and work in Africa. My paper in *Nature* was seen by one Professor George Nelson who, by way of a long chain of interlinked events, led me to set up and run the Schistosomiasis Control Initiative.

But how did I, a boy from Liverpool who had never travelled abroad before, come to be living and working in Africa?

Let's go back a little in time...

1 My Early Years, My Education and My First Job

I was born in the north of England, in York, in 1942, during the Second World War. I lived with my parents in Reighton Avenue, which backed onto an Air Force base, and was therefore a target for enemy bombing raids.

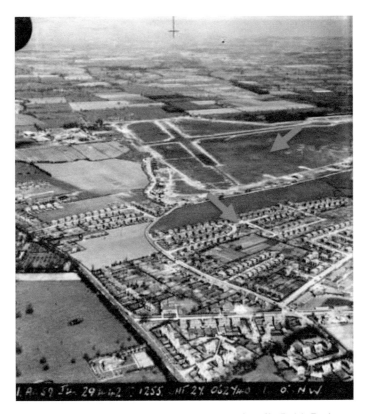

Fig. 1.1. RAF Clifton airfield, York, just after April 1942 Luftwaffe Raid. Red arrow shows my street and the blue arrow the airfield.

© Fenwick, Norris, McCall, 2022. *A Tale of a Man, a Worm and a Snail: The Schistosomiasis Control Initiative* (A. Fenwick *et al.*) DOI: 10.1079/9781786392558.0001

I was told that a neighbour's house received a direct hit but my family home survived.[1] During those difficult war years we hosted some Canadian pilots in our home, and for six years after the war ended, during post-war austerity and food rationing, we received a magnificent food parcel from Canada every Christmas as a thankyou for our hospitality. For my mother's 70th birthday, in 1984, we flew her to Canada to meet those pilots and their families. In 1949, when I was seven years old, my father accepted a job in Sunderland (even further north) and so the family (now with a daughter, Margaret, three years younger than me) moved to this town known for shipbuilding and a football team that played at Roker Park. At the age of 11, I sat, and passed, the 11-plus exam to get into Bede Grammar School in Sunderland, but also passed the entrance exam to the Royal Grammar School in Newcastle. This latter school was recommended to us by a friend of my mother, so this was the one we chose, and I started there in September 1953. I could have been a weekly boarder but we decided that I would be a day pupil. This meant travelling on the steam train every morning from Sunderland to Newcastle at 8.15 am followed by a walk up the hill to Jesmond and to the school. After school we took the 4.15 pm or 4.30 pm train back. There were about eight boys who travelled each day, and the train journey was where I learned how to play bridge, because that was how we passed the time on the train. Sixty-four years later, when I started playing golf midweek in Chalfont St Giles, I played with someone with a Geordie accent (Tim Linton), and as we played we chatted, and worked out that he was one of the boys from the train!

Relocation to Liverpool and Meeting a Beatle or Two

I attended the RGS for just three years because in 1956 we all moved to Liverpool where my father joined Huntley & Palmers (the biscuit maker) as Chief Engineer in their Huyton factory. To have further schooling in the private Merchant Taylors' grammar school, which was the equivalent of the RGS in Newcastle, would have meant a tortuous journey across from south Liverpool, where we lived, to Crosby to the north of Liverpool. Rather than do that, I took up my 11-plus place at the Holt High School in Childwall, just a short cycle ride from our home, which I did every morning. During my two years of the sixth form there, I hooked up with my first girlfriend, who studied at the sister school, Childwall Valley, and we cycled together to and from school every day. We were a strongly linked couple for the whole of our time in the sixth form, and she was a beautiful redhead, a feature that has always attracted me. I guess we moved apart when I went to university, and we lost touch, but I certainly learned a little about relationships – though I still had a lot to learn.

From age 14–18, I did well at school, passing all but one of my O-levels (I failed Woodwork miserably when my practical-test toast rack fell apart!). One highlight of that year was that I shared a weekly lesson on the general paper with John Lennon – (need I say) of Beatles fame – from Quarry Bank

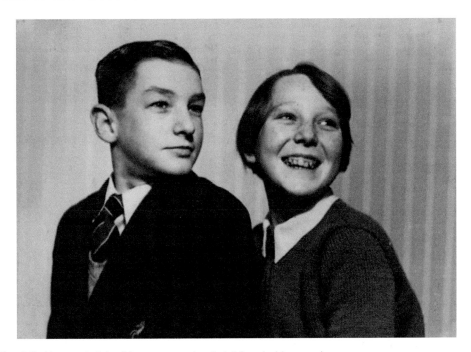

Fig. 1.2. Alan and sister Marney as school children in Liverpool.

School, who was a really funny guy. He became a friend and a member of our 'boys' group'. My lasting memory of him was when our teacher asked us for the major news of the week, expecting the answer that Yuri Gagarin had been shot into space as the first astronaut. John had other ideas and voted for Buddy Holly and the Big Bopper being killed in a plane crash. After my success in my O-levels, I decided on science for the sixth form, where I went on to pass Maths, Physics and Chemistry at A-level, and Maths and Chemistry at S-level, with high-enough marks to earn me the Christopher Bushell Scholarship to Liverpool University. Meanwhile, in the same years, I played a lot of sport – rugby and cricket – for the school, and football for the Woolton St Peter's Church youth club, with friends Peter Bevan, Ian Muir, George Moore and many others. Not only did we play sport together in the club, but we also 'hung out' in Reynolds Park, a small park in Woolton, onto which our house backed. (Incidentally, St Peter's Woolton church youth club was the club that hosted the first-ever meeting of John Lennon and Paul McCartney in 1957 – and I was there!). Subsequently, John, Paul and George Harrison played as a skiffle group and entertained us at our youth club during our evening meetings, with John playing a washboard with thimbles on his fingers and George playing an upturned tea chest with a rope on a pole as a 'double bass'. (There is no need to say what they went on to do – first in Hamburg and then in the UK – while I went to study chemistry at Liverpool University.)

Liverpool University: My Degree in Chemistry

My Introduction to the Performing Arts

Three years later, having worked very hard, attended lectures and done practical laboratory work, I had an honours degree in chemistry, but during those three years I also made some wonderful friends in Peter Hacket, 'Mac' Cowell and David Johnson, and I spent a lot of time with them in a house close to the now-famous Penny Lane. It was during that time that I moved into theatre activities, when I agreed to produce the annual Chemical Society Concert at Liverpool University. Sadly, the society was a bit short of talent that year, so I went along to the local theatre in Hope Street and asked a group, who called themselves the Merseyside Arts Festival Committee, to perform a sketch in the show. They chose to do a skit on *My Fair Lady*, featuring a rather posh lady coming to Liverpool and being taught to speak Scouse. 'I tink she's gorit' was the punch line when the lady could say (in a Scouse accent) 'De girl over thur with the fur hur' and 'De rain in Spain falls mainly on de plain'. The cast in this sketch were, at the time, young unknowns, but they are now all famous in different ways; they included Mike McCartney (Paul's brother), Roger McGough (poet) and John Gorman.[2] Another wonderful defining few weeks for me at Liverpool was when the local golf professional came to the Wednesday university sports afternoon and gave lessons. In three weeks he cured me of the most horrendous 'slice' that I had, so by the time I went to Tanzania I was playing off a 10 handicap!

Enrolling for a PhD at Liverpool School of Tropical Medicine (1963–1966)

After my degree from the chemistry department, I pondered what to study for my PhD and I was introduced to Professor William Kershaw (then Director of Parasitology at the Liverpool School of Tropical Medicine) and Dr Bill Crewe, a senior lecturer at the school. They said they had funding for a research project to determine how effective copper sulphate could be in the control of snails in Africa, and would I, as a chemist, take on the job? The incentive was a three-year contract leading to a PhD and a stipend of £12 a week. I accepted, and moved into a small laboratory/study room at the school in Pembroke Place. The work involved breeding a snail colony and then testing whether copper sulphate would kill these snail species in glass containers, using different concentrations and different exposure times. It did not take long to breed the snails I needed in glass tanks in a warm room, nor to show that in fresh water, in a beaker, the chemical was lethal to snails at low concentrations of 1 part per million. But would the chemical kill snails in African streams and ponds? To answer this question, I altered the contents of the beakers to try to simulate African conditions by using different acidity and alkalinity of the water, by adding a mud layer into the beaker, and then introducing some aquatic plants.

The initial results had been promising, because in the beakers of copper sulphate in clean water, snails succumbed and died quickly. However, in my simulated conditions from Africa, with added mud and plants, the copper sulphate was not as effective. It appeared that the copper sulphate was quickly precipitated as copper carbonate in any alkalinity and was adsorbed in the mud. This meant that the active copper ingredient was removed from contact with the snails and so did not kill them. My three years' PhD research position seemed doomed within three months, because I could not see how the chemical could ever be successful in rural African water bodies. I appeared to have hit a dead end rather quickly.

The Move to Becoming a Parasitologist – a Life-changer

I discussed this rather depressing situation with Bill Crewe and he came up with a compromise solution. He suggested I should do a field research project and write a thesis on parasites of the snails in all the ponds around Liverpool. What a good idea!

Firstly, I did not know there were snails in the Liverpool ponds and certainly was amazed to find them riddled with parasites. I had no idea what species these parasites were, nor did I know, or could guess, what the final host would be. Still, I could try. Once the shape of my MSc thesis was defined, Bill suggested that I should attend some lecture modules (for example, the parasitology lectures designed for doctors studying for a diploma in tropical medicine) and also attend other parasitology lectures by the likes of Dr Clarkson, the veterinary parasitologist at Liverpool, who lectured on parasites of farm animals and pets, and Professor Bill MacDonald, the entomologist at the school, who covered every insect vector that carried the parasites of man and animals.

We cancelled the 'copper' contract but Professor Kershaw kindly promised financial support for one year during which I had to produce an innovative short thesis and pass the exams set for the different modules I had attended. If I was successful, then the school promised it would award me an MSc, so I would not go away empty-handed. This was not an easy task because I was rather short of biology expertise and spent a lot of time learning the names of all these parasites: schistosomiasis, onchocerciasis, the lymphatic filariasis worms *Brugia malayi* and *Wucheraria bancrofti*, tapeworms, and the soil-transmitted helminths (STH) – ascaris, hookworm and trichuris – to name but a few.

While I was struggling with breeding and maintaining a snail colony for my work, I received some unexpected help. One evening, when Professor Kershaw was arriving at Lime Street station after a day in London, he was mugged, and two young students from Canada who witnessed the attack went to his rescue. Sadly, one of the young men was struck by the mugger and lost an eye. After he recovered, Professor Kershaw suggested the students work at the school to earn some money, and one of them was allocated to me. He worked hard for me at a time when I was really quite depressed and rather lazy. For a while, I spent more time across the road following the horses than I spent in the laboratory! That was until I met a beautiful young lady with bright red hair, Julia, and she agreed to be my girlfriend. She worked at the Liverpool School of Tropical Medicine, which allowed us to meet at break- and lunch-times. By then I had a small car, which was fortunate, because she lived the other side of the Mersey and we did spend a lot of time together outside of work. But, sadly, before our relationship could develop, nature intervened. About this time her father died, and she moved away to be with her mother in London, leaving me somewhat broken-hearted. Two years later, unbeknown to me at the time, Julia telephoned me at my office in Tanzania to suggest we get together again, but, sadly, she chose 1 May to phone and the office was closed for the May Day holiday and she did not try again. Three months later I was visiting London so wrote to her to suggest we meet up – but the letter I sent did not reach her until after I had made the visit due to her moving house! So there was no happy ending to this romance and I blame myself for not taking more positive steps to follow up and to foster that relationship.

Unlucky in love, but more fortunate in my science, in 1965 I was awarded an MSc in parasitology and entomology, and my classmate, Sheila, and I were the first students ever to get this degree. Today, both the Liverpool School of Tropical Medicine and the London School of Hygiene and Tropical Medicine award more than 50 MSc degrees in various aspects of parasitology, public health and other related disciplines. We feel proud to have been the 'guinea pigs'.

What to Do with an MSc in Parasitology – Take It to Tanzania

'Wanted: A Biologist with an Interest in Chemistry' (in *Nature*, 1965)

I did wonder what good an MSc in parasitology would be. Well, the wonderful Professor Kershaw had the answer and he called me in to his study to show me an advert in *Nature* journal: 'Wanted: A Biologist with an Interest in Chemistry to research snail control in Arusha in Northern Tanzania'.

'There is no such thing as a biologist with an interest in chemistry who knows anything about snails,' he said, 'so you, as a chemist with an interest in biology and an MSc in snails, will be perfect for the job'.

I applied and was granted an interview in September 1965. The interview was in London, at Eland House, then the home of the Overseas Development Administration (ODA), and I went down on the train to meet three civil servants who looked at my CV and seemed to agree that, indeed, there was no other candidate with any snail experience matching mine. They asked me if I had any questions, which of course I did, but every question I asked about the research institute in Arusha, life there, working conditions and other staff members, were all answered in the same way:

'Well, Mr Fenwick, Dr Hans Hopf should have been on this panel but he withdrew, owing to ill health, at a late stage; he is the expert scientist on our panel and would have been able to answer your questions; we cannot.'

So, I left the interview none the wiser about Arusha and the Tropical Pesticide Research Institute (TPRI). There was no internet or Google in those days.

Admin Cock-up at the ODA

It was at least a month before I received a letter from ODA telling me that I had been successful in my application and was about to be appointed as a Malacologist[3] Research Officer at the TPRI in Arusha (Postal address: PO BOX 3024, Arusha, Tanzania). But, annoyingly, I then heard nothing until the end of January 1966 when I received a letter from ODA saying that the post they had allocated to me had been taken by another candidate, but would I like to go to Arusha as a malaria expert and work on mosquito control? Tempting as this was, because I had nothing else on the horizon, I just felt I had to be honest and decline because I knew so little about mosquitoes and malaria. So what would I do now? I did nothing for a couple of days while I made up my mind. On my 24th birthday, 2 February 1966, I received an airmail letter from Dr Kay Hocking, Director at TPRI, saying, 'Dear Alan, ODA have made their usual cock-up; please be patient while they put things right. We are excited to have you come to TPRI as a snail expert to work on snail control and schistosomiasis control.'

So I waited, and two days later I received yet another letter from ODA: 'Dear Mr Fenwick, having switched a candidate to another vacancy, we are now in a position to offer you the job as Research Officer (Snail Control) at TPRI. Please can you be ready to travel to Arusha on 4 July.'

I accepted the position, thrilled that the contract stated that I would be paid a handsome £1450 per annum, earn 5 days' holiday in the UK for every month I worked, housing would be provided, and if I successfully served my first contract of 21–27 months I would receive a 25% bonus.

My Lifelong Career in Fighting Disease in Africa Begins, 1966

I did all the preparations, vaccinations against yellow fever and cholera, packing a trunk, etc., and waited for my air tickets to arrive – London to Nairobi on a British Airways VC10 and Nairobi to Arusha on an East African Airways DC3, where I would be met by staff from TPRI. The VC10 of course was a narrow plane by today's standards, with three seats either side of one central aisle. It was 'first come, first served' seating in those days and hand luggage had to be placed on an open overhead rack.

I got on the plane early and grabbed a window-seat. The plane filled up until the only seat left was the middle seat next to me. At this point there was a rather loud discussion going on at the door between the airline staff and a tall young man carrying a large double bass. The air hostess repeatedly told him the instrument needed to go in the hold, and he was repeatedly saying 'No way, it is hand luggage'. Eventually, the flight attendants agreed that he could travel with the double bass between his knees. And which seat did he have to take? – the one next to me! He sat down, and, to my amazement, on the cover of the double bass was written the words 'Tropical Pesticides Research Institute, PO Box 3024, Arusha, Tanzania'. I asked if he was working there and he said he was, as an entomologist, specializing in mosquitoes; he was going on a two-year contract to control malaria by killing mosquitoes. (You couldn't make it up!)

'What are you doing there?' he asked, and I replied, 'Research into snails and snail control.'

'How strange,' he said, 'they offered me that job even though I am an entomologist and had applied to research and control mosquitoes! But they switched a candidate to another vacancy and here I am.' ODA efficiency at its best.

This was Jim Hudson, and he and I made it to Arusha where we would share an apartment for two years, working in laboratories next door to each other at TPRI. With this, the story of my work in Africa begins, and that's the story I will now tell.

Notes

1 RAF Clifton was bombed in April 1942.
2 *The Scaffold* consisted of Mike McGear (Mike McCartney), Roger McGough and John Gorman.
3 Someone who studies molluscs.

2 Schistosomiasis and the Amazing Life Cycle of a Killer Worm

My position in TPRI was as a research officer responsible for the study of any or all of the aspects of schistosomiasis. So it's important that I give you a quick tour of the disease, its history and its impact, so that you might understand the state of play when I arrived in Africa in 1966.

Every time a human being, whether a fisherman, a farmer, a housewife, a schoolchild or infant, enters snail-infested fresh water in Africa, they are potentially exposed to minute free-swimming schistosome larvae (cercariae), which can penetrate unbroken skin and begin their trail of destruction through the unfortunate victim's body. Bizarrely, these larvae have come from freshwater snails.

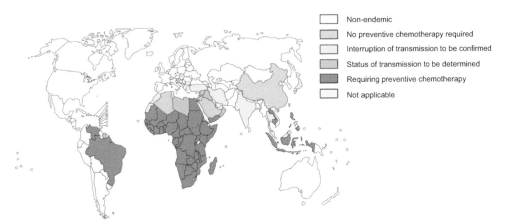

Fig. 2.1. Global distribution of schistosomiasis, 2020. Estimates of the number of people requiring annual preventive chemotherapy were: Africa (211,470,992), Americas (1,620,830), Eastern Mediterranean (20,582,722), South-East Asia (21,815), Western Pacific (2,939,845). (World Health Organization, https://apps.who.int/neglected_diseases/ntddata/sch/sch.html [accessed August 11, 2021].)

© Fenwick, Norris and McCall 2022. *A Tale of a Man, a Worm and a Snail: The Schistosomiasis Control Initiative* (A. Fenwick et al.) DOI: 10.1079/9781786392558.0002

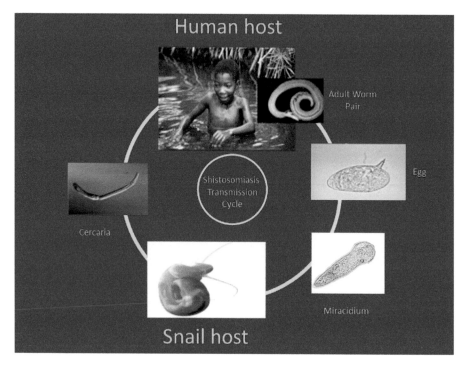

Fig. 2.2. Life cycle of schistosomiasis. (From SCI, adapted by Wendie Norris.)

The Schistosome worm is a parasite that requires two hosts for its reproduction (which is both asexual and sexual). Hosts of the adult worms are always human or animal and there is a mandatory intermediate, asexual, reproductive stage in a species of snail. One species is *Schistosoma haematobium* (*S. haematobium*), which infects people only in Africa and the Middle East and uses *Bulinus* snails as intermediate hosts. A second species found in humans is *S. mansoni,* which was previously only found in Africa but was exported with the slave trade to the Caribbean and South America. This species infects only *Biomphalaria* snails in fresh water. The third species is *S. japonicum*, which is found exclusively in the Far East and uses amphibious *Oncomelania* snails as its intermediate host.

The life cycle and morbidity consequences for the estimated 200 million people infected with one of the three main species of schistosomiasis are mind-blowing.

There are five stages in the life cycle (summarized in Fig. 2.2).

The Stages of the Worm's Life Cycle

Stage 1

An early but rare manifestation of schistosomiasis is nicknamed 'swimmer's itch' and with good reason. This is the effect of the cercariae penetrating the skin in large numbers and causing an allergic reaction at the site of entry. The cercariae attach to the skin with their suckers, burrow into their unsuspecting victim, dropping their forked tail in the process. Once inside, they change from free-swimming larvae into a new form, a schistosomule.

Swimmers itch can also be caused when people bathe in waters with snails harbouring non-human schistosomes: this is a known hazard of swimming in the Great Lakes in North America where, if there is a high-enough density of cercariae searching for wading birds, humans get invaded as well. The cercariae are immediately killed by the human but their death in the skin causes this swimmer's itch.

Stage 2

Once through the skin, the schistosomules take two to three days to enter the underlying blood vessels and get into the circulation from where their journey through the body begins. Their first stop is the lungs where another reaction can take place if large numbers are involved, causing a dry, harsh cough (this is known as Katayama syndrome and used to be very common in Japan and China).

Stage 3

The schistosomules then penetrate the diaphragm to reach the liver where, about one month after entering the human body, they become adult worms growing to a length of about 1 cm, and, having reached maturity, pair off, male and female. The worm pairs then migrate to their preferred blood vessels where they settle and live for several years. The blood vessel site depends on the species of parasite: *S. mansoni* prefers the veins of the intestine and *S. haematobium* migrates to those of the bladder.

Stage 4

The adult worms remain inside the blood vessels, living off the blood, and the female worms lay their eggs, as many as 300 per day (sexual reproduction). The eggs are swept away in the bloodstream but for the cycle to be completed they need to leave the human body to reach fresh water, hatch and infect the host snails. Many eggs do get out (*S. haematobium* eggs via the bladder and urine and *S. mansoni* eggs through the intestine and faeces) but many do not and it is these eggs trapped in the bladder wall or swept to the liver that cause long-term damage to the human host. In both sites, the bladder wall and the liver, the trapped eggs die and evoke a response from the immune system which leads to millions of minute scars and eventually fibrosis and blockage of the organs involved. Thus, contrary to popular belief, it is in fact the eggs and not the worms which cause most of the clinical symptoms of schistosomiasis.

Stage 5

If the eggs do break out from the blood vessels and reach either the bladder or intestine, they will be excreted to continue with their fight for survival. How do they break out? How do they reach the snails in river water?

The eggs of *S. haematobium* sport a cutting device on one end, and as such are known as terminal-spined eggs, which operate like tin-openers slicing their way through the bladder wall, releasing eggs and blood and turning the urine red as they go. Both stools and urine will contain blood from the broken blood vessels. It's the bloody stool and especially the more obvious blood in the urine ('red wee') that are the early symptoms of schistosomiasis infection and are a definitive diagnosis in children. The swollen bellies are late symptoms.

In rural villages where there are no toilet facilities, people urinate and defecate in streams or on the banks of streams and other water bodies. The eggs are thus washed into the water where they can hatch. The emerging larvae (called miracidia) have a short, free-swimming life, maybe less than eight hours, in which to find a snail of the correct species to penetrate. If they do succeed in finding their correct snail, asexual development takes place. Over a period of a month, the miracidia develop into sporocysts which, in turn, produce a generation of daughter sporocysts inside which cercariae are formed.

When the asexual reproduction is complete, the next-stage larvae (cercariae) emerge from the snail as free-swimming larvae to seek out a human host (see stage 1) and complete the cycle. Meanwhile, the poor snail has been taken over by the parasite and becomes a production line for thousands of cercariae for as long as it continues to live.

An Amazing Life Cycle

What an amazing life cycle! The schistosome worm belongs to a group of helminth worms called 'trematodes' (or flukes) who all have this unique way of life: male and female worms live in one host and their eggs need to develop asexually in a specific snail species. Some trematodes infect only humans, and others infect non-human hosts – e.g. wading birds, cattle, sheep and rodents; each trematode species has its own snail!

Thus, it takes at least two months for the human schistosomiasis cycle to be completed, from an egg being laid in a human host to the next generation of an adult worm laying eggs in another new host. I continuously ask myself how did the life cycle develop?

In effect, schistosomiasis is a by-product of the way people in rural communities lived their daily lives, depending on natural water bodies for all uses, including sanitation. Transmission depends on people urinating and defecating in and near to the ponds, lakes, streams and rivers where they also wash and bathe. Another behaviour that assists the schistosome to proliferate is the use of 'night soil' (i.e. faeces) as a fertilizer in irrigated fields, a practice particularly common in the Far East, because this spreads the schistosome eggs and allows them to hatch and infect snails.

The life cycle is, however, so precarious that the chance of any one egg becoming an adult worm is infinitesimal. But the reproduction potential is massive because the urine or faeces of an infected individual can harbour hundreds or thousands of eggs which, if deposited in fresh water, hatch into those free-swimming miracidia whose sole purpose is to seek out a snail host to continue with the next stage of the life cycle; a complicated but successful strategy. As humans have survived and populations have grown, the schistosomes have proliferated and will continue to do so until socio-economic development and better hygiene reduce the chances of eggs reaching snails.

The Cercariae 'Cloaking' Device

How do the cercariae, which get into the human body, avoid detection by our immune system when they transform into schistosomules and migrate through to the lung and liver to become mature worms? Somehow, they evade our defences, and we now know that they quickly disguise themselves with human antigen, making themselves invisible to the host's immune system (an 'invisibility cloak', if you will) (see Chapter 17).

Considering that the adult worms may live in the human body for between five and 20 years, and each female can lay up to 300 eggs per day, the potential for both infecting the environment and getting trapped in the human body is enormous.

The First Discovery of the Live Adult Worm in Man in 1852

Despite having parasitized man for millennia, the adult schistosome worm was first seen and its importance realized as recently as 1852 during *post mortem* examinations in Egypt. Theodore Maximilian Bilharz, a German physician, discovered *S. haematobium* as the cause of urinary (now known as uro-genital) schistosomiasis when carrying out an autopsy in Cairo, but he had no idea of the involvement of snails, and he did not work out the stages of transmission. Neither did he realize that there were two very similar African species. It then took over 60 years from this, the first published definition of the adult worm, for someone (credited to Robert Leiper, 1915) to decipher the obligatory African snail participation in the life cycle.

The snail connection was first established in studies with the Asian species of schistosomiasis, *S. japonicum,* conducted by Miyairi and Suzuki

(1913), so Leiper knew what to look for. Clearly stamping his mark in the history of schistosomiasis, Leiper confirmed two separate snail hosts, one each for *S. mansoni* (Biomphalaria) and *S. haematobium* (Bulinus). Thus, at last we had the life cycle of the parasite which caused a disease about which little was known, other than it was considered to be 'perhaps the most dreadful of the remaining plagues of Egypt' (Madden, 1910).

In contrast, unravelling the life cycle of Asiatic schistosomiasis described in Katayama, Japan, in 1847 by Yoshinao Fujii – there being only one species in the region – had been relatively straightforward in comparison to the African forms of disease.

The *Bulinus* and *Biomphalaria* snails, vital to the schistosome life cycle in Africa, both thrive in freshwater bodies in tropical climates and thrive in areas frequented by man. In fact, they are in abundance, possibly because they favour environments rich in human excreta and the detritus of everyday living. They tend to live most of their lives in one small habitat but can be carried by freshwater currents or possibly water birds from one water body to another. However, it is rarely the snails that are responsible for dispersal of the parasite; this is a role usually reserved for the human host. In my lectures I was taught that schistosomiasis is 'a disease of snails carried by small boys'.

Early attempts at control

In the early 20th century, because no effective drug was available and the snail was an essential host in the schistosome life cycle, it was considered that the snail was surely the prime target for control. 'No snails, no transmission' was the target.

Once he understood the life cycle, and involvement of two separate parasites and host snails, Leiper began looking for methods of control. Knowing full well that it would be near-impossible to prevent water contamination, he initially explored methods to kill cercariae with sodium bisulphate and for controlling the snail population. He also made recommendations such as drawing water from deep wells or, if surface water had to be used, then intake pipes should draw from the 'centre of the stream and should draw water from near the bottom and at a place where there is little vegetation'. This indicated his thorough knowledge of the distribution of snails near to the water's edge.

Several chemicals or 'molluscicides; have been used over the years to try to kill off the snails and prevent transmission (including copper sulphate, which was the first to be used – and hence my employment to study its use). Over the years, biological control using either predators or competitor species, and environmental manipulation of the habitat (draining swamps, etc.) have also been considered, but these methods have never really proved effective except in small specialist sites. The snail reproduces extremely quickly and has an amazing power to survive.

Many of Leiper's environmental control measures, such as locating roads and villages on irrigation schemes away from canals, are as relevant now as they were 100 years ago. However, one considerable change in approach to control methods is evident today which Leiper dismissed out of hand: he failed to engage local communities in overcoming the disease. His methods focused on the killing of snails rather than how to control a disease in the population. Snail control was not finally superseded by medical interventions until the 1980s when the new drug praziquantel became available. This was the first acceptable drug with a better cure rate and fewer side-effects than earlier drugs. The changeover was also made because the snails had proved extremely difficult to kill, and the chemicals used were expensive and environmentally unacceptable.

During the period 1950–1980, several drugs were tested and after positive initial results they were marketed to treat schistosomiasis. These included metrifonate, oxamniquine, hycanthone and niridazole, but each drug turned out to have either serious side-effects or insufficient efficacy, or resistance developed, and so these proved not to be commercially viable.

The SCI's success (more about this later) has been largely due to an updated approach, namely a combination of the availability of an effective chemotherapy (praziquantel) and active participation in improving water and sanitation by local communities.

A Disease with a Long History in Egypt

Alarmingly, despite the considerable medical advances of our age, some diseases still manage to remain as virulent today as they were thousands of years ago. Records suggest that the uro-genital form of schistosomiasis caused by *S. haematobium* has been around since the days of ancient Egypt (3150–30 BC). We know this because the naturally dry environment and preservation techniques of mummification by the Egyptian civilization have allowed us to recover schistosome eggs (with their separate distinctive spines) from ancient Egyptian mummies. There is also reference to the worms and the voiding of blood in urine in hieroglyphic writings which refer to haematuria or *weseh* in the papyrus of Kahun and of Ebres (Jordan and Webbe, 1993).

Scholars are divided over the accuracy of references to eggs and worms in medical papyri, but the paleopathological evidence derived from mummified tissue is far more convincing. In 1910, the calcified eggs of *Bilharzia haematobium*, as the disease was then known, were found in the kidney tubules of Egyptian mummies of the 20th Dynasty (Ruffer, 1910). Almost 90 years later, this was supported by the discovery of schistosome eggs in the poorly preserved kidneys of Nakht, the mummy of a teenage boy. In the same mummy, calcified eggs were found in the portal area where an artery links the liver and intestines (Nunn and Tapp, 2000).

In modern Egypt, in the 1920s, it was recognized that schistosomiasis was a disease that needed to be controlled, and a long-standing elimination programme began, finally achieving success when an extensive national treatment programme with praziquantel was conducted from 1989 to 2002 (see later). Throughout the 20th century, squamous cell carcinoma of the bladder (caused by long-term infection with uro-genital schistosomiasis) was the country's leading cause of cancer, but by 2000 it was gradually disappearing, and since 2015 it has been virtually unknown. This achievement stands as testament to the success of removing the potentially lethal effects of the worm and its eggs.

Red Wee and Swollen Bellies – Symptoms and Consequences

Schistosomiasis is a destructive disease but the damage to organs is usually noticed only after the accumulation of very high numbers of worms and eggs. In individuals with fewer worms, symptoms may not become apparent for many years. In other individuals exposed to water with a high concentration of cercariae, or who have repeatedly entered the same contaminated body of water, symptoms become obvious more quickly. On occasions, in exceptionally heavy transmission conditions, severe disease has been known to kill people within two months.

As a general rule, in untreated communities, studies have shown that both intensity and prevalence of disease as measured by eggs in excreta, peak in 10- to 14-year-old children before the egg output drops off, but of course undiagnosed damage to internal organs can be insidiously continuing through adulthood.

The symptoms of the two forms found in Africa have some common clinical features in early stages but the consequences of advanced disease manifest very differently.

Uro-genital schistosomiasis

The classic symptom is blood in the urine ('red wee').

It has been estimated that the mean output of eggs per *S. haematobium* pair is approximately 20 times greater than the egg output of *S. mansoni*. Thus, many more *S. haematobium* eggs fail to get into the bladder and out of the body, but will be trapped in the bladder wall. When these eggs die, they cause 'sandy-coloured patches', lesions, ulcers and granulomas (small nodules of inflammatory cells). Calcification and fibrosis occur. *S. haematobium* is the major cause of 'calcified bladder', with up to 100,000 eggs/cm^2 of tissue. Bladder neck fibrosis leads to reduced bladder function. Later-stage infections may show black calcified eggs in the urine, and are linked to bladder cancer.

S. haematobium can cause female genital schistosomiasis (because dying eggs can produce lesions on the cervix) leading to infertility and an increased

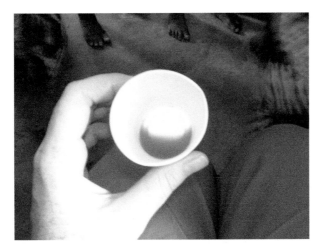

Fig. 2.3. Bloody urine sample.

risk of contracting HIV when young women become sexually active. An under-reported and often misdiagnosed aspect of the disease, it is estimated to affect over 56 million African women and girls (Kjetland *et al.*, 2008).

Intestinal schistosomiasis

In contrast to uro-genital disease, intestinal schistosomiasis caused by *S. mansoni* takes a different course: early symptoms (acute disease) are bloody stools containing many eggs. This is because the worms reside in the blood vessels around the intestine and their escape route to the outside world is thus in the stools. The passage of eggs through the intestine may vary from day to day and can even self-limit with abdominal symptoms (bloody stool, intermittent diarrhoea and discomfort – feeling full) disappearing within three months of onset, without treatment.

Chronic disease due to *S. mansoni* has an altogether more complicated picture. The eggs which fail to leave the body are either trapped in the intestine wall or are swept back into the liver, via the hepatic portal system. From the liver they have nowhere to go, and so eventually there is an accumulation of dead eggs, and the inevitable immune response leads to inflammation (a granuloma forms around each egg to isolate it) and minute scars (fibrosis). The ever-increasing numbers of eggs produce more fibrosis, then calcification, and finally cirrhosis in the worst cases. As the process continues, the patient's abdomen becomes tender, and the liver enlarged and hardened. Eventually the liver's blood supply is physically obstructed.

Most patients will accommodate for the reduced blood flow with an increase in artery supply but in severe cases, the fibrotic liver will induce hypertension, and fluid accumulates to give the sufferer the characteristic 'swollen belly'. As this stage worsens, the patient may suffer a gastric

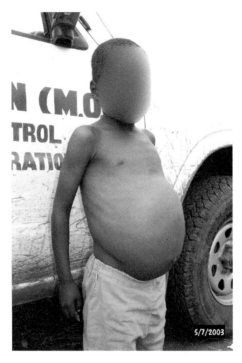

Fig. 2.4. Boy with swollen belly due to S. mansoni infection.

haemorrhage and bleed from their mouth. Sadly, little can be done at this advanced stage of the disease and death may be inevitable.

An Invisible, Silent and Deadly Enemy

But despite these horrific long-term effects, many individuals with schistosomiasis are unaware of the silent turmoil going on beneath the surface. They are usually oblivious to any damage occurring to their liver until the disease is well advanced or the shock of vomiting blood awakens them to their predicament.

Thus, schistosomiasis can kill, and the generally offered estimate is that it claims the lives of around 280,000 people, annually, worldwide, a highly significant number especially for an easily preventable disease. But we have no real evidence as to whether this estimate is accurate and it may well have been much higher during the period 1960–2000 before widespread treatment programmes began. Accurate figures for deaths and cause of deaths in these under-resourced communities just do not exist. Also, where records are kept, deaths from liver disease and bleeding from varices are not always attributed to an earlier schistosomiasis infection.

Most patients live but are left with chronic ill health which so weakens them that they may be unable to perform simple daily activities or work. In children, enlargement of the liver may retard physical growth, and in adults, hormonal changes may interfere with the reproductive system causing amenorrhea (absence of menstruation in females), early menopause, infertility and loss of libido. In some countries, the return of libido in men served as the best motivator for adult compliance when rumours (unconfirmed) spread that praziquantel was an aphrodisiac.

Sufferers of either or both schistosome species (and STH, as they often occur together) thus may experience diarrhoea, abdominal pain, blood in stool, stunted growth, anaemia due to blood loss, exercise intolerance and reduced cognitive function (King *et al.*, 2005; Koukounari *et al.*, 2006).

But in Africa, where almost everyone has parasites, what is normal? If the symptoms start at an early age, then sufferers may not know what it was like to be fit and healthy, and so do not recognize their ill-health. Red wee was, in the past, even seen as a 'rite of passage' for young boys.

3 Coming of Age in Tanzania – Arusha, 1966–1971

My new research post at TPRI had, in the recent past, been the province of Ray Foster and Norman Crossland, both prolific researchers who each went on to work in UK pharmaceutical companies Pfizer and Shell, respectively, and contribute to the development of new products for schistosomiasis control (the drug oxamniquine,[1] which preceded praziquantel as a treatment for *S. mansoni*, and the molluscide Frescon, which held promise for some time until being superseded by Bayluscide).

I had a lot to live up to.

I spent the next five years in Arusha, initially researching how to kill snails using different chemicals, first in the laboratory and then in a small field plot consisting of five canals provided by the Tanganyika Planting Company (TPC) on a sugar estate a few miles from Moshi. Arusha is situated at the foot of Mount Meru, the second-highest mountain in Tanzania, and Moshi some 50 km away at the foot of the highest mountain in Africa, Mount Kilimanjaro.

Much of equatorial Africa's enduring appeal lies in its unfettered display of rich and unruly flora and fauna and its diversity of human culture. I drove that tarmac road from Arusha to Moshi and back at least twice a week, on every journey marvelling at the landscape and the free-roaming game. Every wild animal in Africa seemed to be just on the side of the road – lions, cheetahs, wildebeest, many Thompsons and Grant gazelles and giraffes. Once I watched a mongoose and a snake fight a duel in the middle of the road. Today, between the same two towns, there is an international airport (Kilimanjaro Airport) and a densely populated strip of land with not a gazelle to be seen.

The TPRI management allowed me a free hand to conduct research into any aspects of schistosomiasis and so I diversified and moved on to investigate the epidemiology of schistosomiasis, tested new drugs (for treating people (Fenwick, 1971)) as well as new molluscicides (Fenwick, 1969; Fenwick and Lidgate, 1970). I carried out cost-benefit analyses of treatments to identify the financial cost to sugarcane-cutters of their being less productive due to infection (Fenwick, 1972a; Fenwick and Figenschou, 1972). Finally, in conjunction with the resident doctor at TPC, we attempted to reduce the prevalence of the disease and the suffering it caused to the people on the sugar estate (Fenwick, 1972b; Fenwick and Jorgennesen, 1972).

Death of My Father

It was at this time (1967), during my first tour in Tanzania, whilst I was working away from Arusha on a field trip, that three telegrams arrived for me in succession at TPRI. On my return I found that my mother had written that my father was ill and in hospital, then that he had to have an operation to remove his gall bladder, and finally that he had died during the operation. I managed to telephone home to learn that he had already been cremated. My mother and sister said there was no point in me flying back as I was due to go on leave shortly afterwards; so, sadly, I was never able to say goodbye to my father.

Tanzania was life-changing for me on so many fronts: I fell in love with all aspects of East Africa, from its plant life on Mount Kilimanjaro to the wild animals in the game parks, to the uniqueness of the Tanzanian Masai and the Chaga tribes. I was fascinated. I met and married my first wife, Irene in 1968. I took up Scottish dancing, got hooked on amateur dramatics with the group who performed at Arusha's Little Theatre and had some really good fortune with a study I carried out into bilharzia infections in wild baboons.

Marriage Beckons and Child Number 1 Arrives

I met Irene, a teacher at Arusha School, on an organized climb of about 12 people to the summit of Kilimanjaro. After the climb, we courted and visited the game parks together and attended weekly Scottish dancing lessons. Finally, we married in August 1968 in Arusha church, and my best man was Donough Mahon, son of a coffee farmer whose family had befriended me. I moved out of the flat I was sharing with Jim Hudson and was allocated a house in Barabara ya Serengeti where we lived until we left Arusha in 1971. Our first daughter, Janet, was born in September 1969 in Nairobi and enjoyed a happy infancy in Arusha.

Arusha: A Blend of Culture and the Caledonian Ball

In Africa there are many different cultures; some we understand but some retain that element of mystery. Negotiations follow a different code of practice and very distinctive etiquette. One of my favourite memories of African humour occurred in Arusha in 1968.

We spent every Tuesday evening at Tengeru Club, practising Scottish dancing for the annual event of the year, the Caledonian Ball, on 30 November. There were not that many Scots in Arusha, but those that were there were more 'Scottish than the Scots', and they jealously guarded their right to buy a table for eight at the Caledonian Ball and form a group that would dance.

One day, a Tanzanian gentleman and his wife turned up and asked if they might join the dancing class. Alex Nyrenda worked for the Shell Oil company, and was actually famous locally because he was the Tanzanian citizen selected to plant the national flag on the top of Mount Kilimanjaro at independence in 1961, when he was in the army. They were very likeable and mixed in well at the classes. When the time came for booking tables for the event, Alex asked the chieftain of the St Andrew's Society whether he might book a table for himself and some friends. This seemed like it might be an embarrassing question, since the rule was very strictly adhered to that only Scots were allowed that privilege. The chieftain was acutely aware of the embarrassment but felt he had to say that only Scots could book tables. Alex saved the moment quite brilliantly by stating that he had Scottish blood in him.

'Really?' said the relieved chieftain.

'Yes indeed,' said Alex with a straight face, 'my grandfather once ate a Scottish missionary.'

Problem solved with a hint of humour, and Alex was granted leave to buy a table.

Other enjoyable pastimes and highlights of the social life in Arusha, were playing golf (evenings and weekends) and participating in the Little Theatre, first as an actor and then in stage management. In my last year in Tanzania I had watched Clive Rushbrooke, headmaster of the Arusha School and a talented theatrical director, write and direct a pantomime in which I acted. I was so taken with this that I determined to copy his ideas at my next opportunity.

Life was not all fun, however, for expats; it could be scary. In 1969 there was an outbreak of bubonic plague at Arusha hospital, starting with two infected farmworkers brought into the town from an outlying farm, which led to them and five hospital staff dying and the whole of Arusha town being put into quarantine for two weeks. It was necessary for East African Airways to fly a plane over and drop sulphadimidine tablets for us all to take.

Trips to the Game Parks

The most attractive part of Tanzania is the game parks. I became good friends with Ian Douglas Hamilton (the elephant zoologist whose infection with bilharzia led to my *Nature* paper [see Prologue]) and stayed with him often at Lake Manyara. I took many photographs of lions in trees, rhinos and elephants, to name but a few. The bird life was incredible. From Lake Manyara I went on to the unique Ngorongo crater and further still to the Leakey sites of the first human settlements at Olduvai Gorge and to the Serengeti where I saw my first wild leopard.

We were just so lucky to be there in the late sixties because at that time there were so few tourists that one did not need to stick to the roads to view the animals. Today, with radios between the many vehicles, and so many tourists, finding animals and watching them is not quite the adventure it was.

Professor George Nelson Affected My Life Journey

Let me refer back to my earlier story of baboons at Lake Manyara and introduce you to Professor George Nelson. Meeting George changed my life. It
was 1970, my five-year contract at TPRI was coming to an end and I had been
invited to attend the African Union health conference in Addis Ababa. On
my way to Arusha airport to catch my flight, I picked up my mail from the
post office and found a letter from London. It was from George, asking me if
I would be interested in working in Sudan for the Wellcome Trust, because he
had just awarded two PhDs to Mutamad Ahmed El Amin and Abdel Hamid
Sayed Omer.

Professor Nelson wanted them to return to Sudan and work in the
Ministry of Health and the university, respectively, but he felt they needed
external support with someone to work with them on research and control of
schistosomiasis in Sudan. I was not too sure but could not argue with the turn
of events because when I arrived in Addis Ababa for the meeting, Professor
Nelson was there and so was Mutamad. Also there was Dick Pearce from
Shell Chemicals, Khartoum. Shell had just formulated a new molluscicide,
N-trityl morpholine (Frescon), and were very interested to find someone to
test the product in the field. They thought that I might be the right person
to do so and Sudan might be the right place. Dick Pearce offered to divert
me through Khartoum on my way back to Arusha and provided me with an

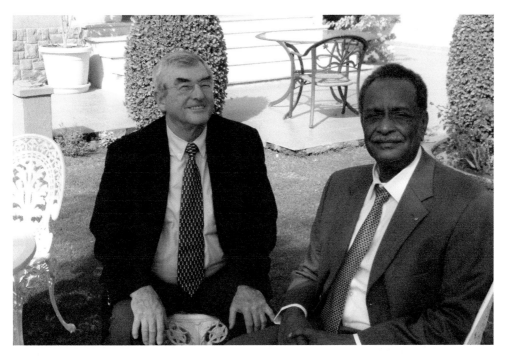

Fig. 3.1. With Mutamad Ahmed El Amin.

air ticket from Addis Ababa to Khartoum and then back to Arusha to see if I could be tempted. The offer included luxurious accommodation and I *was* tempted! I accepted his offer.

There was one condition, however – I had to have submitted my PhD thesis to the Liverpool School of Tropical Medicine and have it awarded before I could go to Khartoum. So with the help of my supervisor, Professor Bill MacDonald, I spent four months in early 1971 working at the Liverpool school completing my thesis. Liverpool selected Professor George Nelson to be the external examiner at my *viva voce* exam! He gave me a hard time but I passed, and so I could set off for Khartoum. The PhD thesis included several publications in top peer-reviewed journals covering topics like snail-control experiments, the efficacy of some medications, the baboon work, cost-effective treatments and the success of mass drug treatments in the sugar estate, a study in the economic cost of infections, plus snail-control trials in canals.

1966–1971 in Summary

To summarize, I had left the UK in 1966 as an inexperienced and unknown young man with energy, enthusiasm and some scientific knowledge and returned a different person. By early 1971, after five years in Tanzania, I had gained some international standing, managed a team of technicians, published five papers in the *Bulletin of the World Health Organization* on different aspects of schistosomiasis and published a ground-breaking paper on baboon infections in the *Transactions of the Royal Society of Tropical Medicine and Hygiene*. I was married, with a daughter and enough money in the bank to buy our first house. I had enough research results to complete a PhD, a promise of an exciting position funded by the Wellcome Trust in the London School of Hygiene and Tropical Medicine (LSHTM), and the opportunity to continue working on schistosomiasis abroad, this time in Sudan.

I went to Khartoum a wiser person, full of energy and wanting to make my mark in the scientific community, and ten years' worth of funding from the trust with which to do it.

Note

[1] Oxamniquine derivatives have now been developed which treat all forms of human schistosomiasis and are being explored to deal with praziquantel resistance (multidrug therapy) (Guzman *et al.*, 2020).

4 Research, Training and Drug Testing in Sudan, 1971–1988

Preparing Sudan's Young Medical Students

I think that everyone I have told is totally amazed that someone could live and work in Sudan for what turned out to be 17 years. Sudan was recognized as an extreme-hardship post, but I just loved the time I spent there conducting research on schistosomiasis, training and working closely with local staff, testing new drugs and molluscicides, and writing publications with my Sudanese colleagues, particularly Dr Mutamad Ahmed El Amin and Dr Abdel Hamid Sayed Omer. Irene and I found a small house to rent and we employed an Ethiopian lady, Zaudi, to be a 'nanny' for our daughter Janet. Zaudi had a young son, Joseph, who came to live with us, and he and Janet became great friends.

My funding from Harvard-Wellcome was initially for ten years, and it also came with an appointment as a Wellcome Fellow in Professor Nelson's department at LSHTM.

I was based in Khartoum at the Stack Laboratories, in the Schistosomiasis Research and Control Department on the fifth floor. The building belonged to the Ministry of Health and was situated in front of the City Hospital and opposite the railway station, looking in one direction, and the Gordon School of Medicine in the other.

The ambition of every educated Sudanese school boy and girl was to become a doctor, and the School of Medicine – the only one in the country in 1971 – enrolled the top 100 students from the various secondary schools every year. When I first arrived and took on some teaching responsibilities, the trainees were mostly male, but as time passed, this changed. All the secondary schools dotted around the country were boarding schools and, of course, there was no mixing of boys and girls. More girls' schools were opened and more girls received a secondary education. The consequence of these schools was that the girls were very carefully chaperoned and were not allowed any freedom after school hours, and so they worked at their homework. The boys' schools, meanwhile, allowed their pupils much more freedom and in the villages the pupils could be seen after school roaming around, drinking tea in cafés and playing football, but not working as hard as the girls. It was not too long before the top 100 being admitted to the School of Medicine became unbalanced, with

© Fenwick, Norris and McCall 2022. *A Tale of a Man, a Worm and a Snail: The Schistosomiasis Control Initiative* (A. Fenwick *et al.*) DOI: 10.1079/9781786392558.0004

a higher percentage of the intake being female. These ladies were incredibly bright and became well-educated doctors. But this posed a problem.

In Sudan almost every town had a small hospital, described as a 'one-doctor hospital', and traditionally, the newly graduated doctors would be allocated to a hospital for two years where they learned their trade living in rather sparse quarters in the hospital. While this was fine for male graduates, it did not go down very well with the parents of female graduates as the traditions in Sudan expected females to marry and have children at the end of their education. To meet the demand for doctors in the rural towns, some changes were needed, and the School of Medicine partly tackled this problem by limiting the intake to 50% male and 50% female. Teaching these medical students became an enjoyable sideline for me.

Killing Snails and Curing People

Molluscides and brown beans

The first few years in Sudan were spent testing Shell's molluscicide Frescon (N-trityl morpholine) to see if it would eliminate snails in small ditches, streams and ponds near villages and then testing Frescon and Bayluscide (niclosamide, produced by Bayer) in the vast network of canals in the Gezira scheme. (This scheme lay between the Blue and White Niles to the south of Khartoum and its 100% prevalence rate for schistosomiasis was the main reason for my posting in 1971.) It was incredibly frustrating that Frescon was lethal to snails in the laboratory, but in any moving water the snails just refused to go. Part of the problem was that Frescon did not kill snail eggs and so re-population was rapid (Amin *et al.*, 1976).

We carried out many field experiments using different application techniques and dosages, and after each field trial I would take the field technicians and snail collectors for a breakfast in our village called Meilig. We always frequented the same café and ordered full breakfasts of boiled brown beans with onions, goat's cheese and oil, and then liver fried with onions. After one particularly large group of 15 delivered his biggest payday ever, the café owner took to grinning at me as soon as he saw me arrive. He nicknamed me Mia Talata wa Hamseen [Arabic for 153] because the bill for the breakfast was one pound 53 piastres – literally about £1.50 for 15 people! Things were very reasonably priced in rural Sudan in the 1970s.

In the Gezira canals, we concluded, in 1979, that Bayluscide was more effective than Frescon in reducing the snail population for longer periods (Amin and Fenwick, 1977). We tried different methods of applying the chemicals to the canals – drip feeding, knapsack spraying, and then moved on to large-scale aerial spraying (Amin and Fenwick, 1975). Each had their merits and drawbacks – drip feeding would not work in slow-moving or stagnant water and knapsack spraying was impractical because there were so many canals. Aerial spraying had been used in West Africa against black flies (the vector for *Onchocerca*, which causes river blindness). This proved to

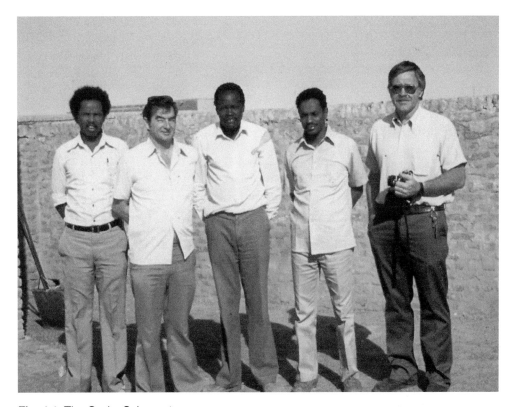

Fig. 4.1. The Gezira Scheme team.

be rather hazardous for the crop-spraying pilot flying low over the canals, though exciting to watch, but the real drawback for our project was the cost. We also conducted prevalence studies (Omer *et al.*, 1976).

Then, in the early 1970s, praziquantel appeared as a promising drug against schistosomiasis and Professor Amin, Dr Said Omer and I were asked by WHO to test the drug in an experimental setting in the Gezira Scheme.

Field trials of praziquantel

We designed a study and selected the village of Angado in the northern Gezira (with the approval of the sheikh of the village). Every resident provided a stool sample, and we examined these and randomly divided the positives into two groups. One group was treated with praziquantel, 40 mg/kg body weight, after breakfast and the second group with 20 mg/kg in the morning after breakfast, followed by another 20 mg/kg in the afternoon, again after food. Everyone was followed up with stool-sample examinations regularly over a 12-month period and the cure rates and egg count reductions in each group calculated (Kardaman *et al.*, 1983).

To carry out this study, we needed the collaboration, co-operation and compliance of everyone enrolled in the study, and for this I enlisted the help of a social anthropologist named Ann Allen who taught at Khartoum University. She helped me recruit a young village resident, Awatif, who spoke some English. Employing Awatif was very helpful to her and her family because her father (the village bus driver) had a long-term illness and was being treated in Omdurman and staying with relatives there. One Thursday, when I was about to drive back to my family in Khartoum, Awatif asked if she could come with me so that she could visit her father. I insisted on taking her to her father's residence even though it was the other side of the river. Of course, then I had to go into the house to greet them all and they persuaded me to stay for a meal (typical Sudanese hospitality). I sat with her father and chatted to him. The poor man was obviously weak and tired, not to mention unhappy at being unable to drive and therefore earn money for the family. He thought I was a doctor, I think, because he insisted on showing me his medical records which were all in English and he did not know what they said. Before I could finish reading, the meal arrived, and in typical Sudanese fashion we both ate from the same bowl using our hands. After the meal I finished reading his records and came to the final diagnosis which was leprosy – ooops! He was being treated with dapsone, which does not work for everyone and causes side-effects, and, clearly, he was not getting better.

When I got home, I quickly researched leprosy (not wanting to succumb myself) and was pleased to find that dapsone would render him not infective to others. Leprosy is curable, and I read about a new treatment, rifampicin (now a standard), and as dapsone wasn't working well, I managed to get him some rifampicin. When he took it, the recovery was amazing, and within a month he was back in the village driving his bus. I became a hero and was welcomed in the village every time I went there, and compliance with our drug trial was almost 100%.

My timing was great – being asked to do these field tests of praziquantel – for as a result of this and other trials it became available for widespread use in the 1980s, and it has gone on to be the drug of choice.

Praziquantel, the wonderdrug

Praziquantel was initially developed for the veterinary market.

During the 1970s, two German pharmaceutical companies, Bayer and E. Merck, collaborated in trials to confirm the compound's curative properties against various worms that were pathogenic to man, and schistosomes were found to be the most responsive to treatment. (More about this in Chapter 15.)

To demonstrate praziquantel's safety and efficacy, Bayer approached the World Health Organization (WHO) to request collaboration in multi-centre clinical trials. My long-time friend and mentor Dr Andrew Davis (who sadly died at the age of 84 in January 2013) co-ordinated these. As a result, from 1973, when praziquantel was first patented until one decade later, more than

400 articles were published on the pre-clinical and clinical aspects of the new product. During this period, praziquantel was used for safe and effective treatment in over 25,000 patients on three continents. Repeat trials, clinical experience and large-scale field control programmes all confirmed it was exceptionally safe, efficacious and cheap to use, and it was cleared for use in mass drug administration (MDA) programmes. There has been little evidence of resistance developing even after many millions of treatments being dispensed.

Despite the relative simplicity and effectiveness of the annual praziquantel 'swallow-and-go' regimen, the task of making this drug available to the many communities in need in Africa has proved to be an uphill struggle.

100 Years of De-worming

But before praziquantel became available, was schistosomiasis being treated? We need to return to the end of the First World War – prior to 1920 – when a scientist based in Egypt reported the first successful treatment of schistosomiasis using antimony potassium tartrate. In fact, at the time, Dr J.B. Christopherson had been using the antimony-based drugs to treat leishmaniasis, a parasitic disease transmitted by sandflies, which causes horrible skin ulcers and can invade internal organs, with fatal consequences. Christopherson noticed that those patients co-infected with *S. haematobium* and suffering from blood in their urine, stopped peeing blood (Christopherson, 1919). A medication to cure schistosomiasis had been discovered.

Consequently, the first known treatment control programmes were carried out against schistosomiasis in Egypt and Sudan, particularly targeting the Egyptian labourers – of which there were thousands – who migrated to the Sudan to dig the water channels for the Gezira irrigation scheme.

Despite these antimonial compounds being unpleasantly toxic, and the necessity for 14 consecutive daily injections to effect a cure, the regimen was used for many years as the only available treatment. Several decades later, in the 1950s and 60s, came the next generation of drugs – without antimony – namely niridazole, hycanthone, metrifonate and oxamniquine, each of which was used in a range of campaigns. The largest campaign was probably in the heavily infected Fayoum irrigation project in Egypt in the late 70s. But as these drugs became more widely used, unacceptable adverse events emerged – psychotic reactions to niridazole and deaths due to liver complications after hycanthone (Fenwick *et al.*, 2003).

The best of these drugs was metrifonate, which was inexpensive and effective against *S. haematobium* in Africa, but only when the complicated regimen of three treatments given a week apart was adhered to. This triple treatment made compliance an obstacle for mass drug administration programmes. Oxamniquine proved to be effective against *S. mansoni* (but only on the adult worms) and was used in South America, the Caribbean and West Africa. It was used extensively in Brazil until reports of resistance (reviewed in Chevalier *et al.*, 2019).

Thus, when praziquantel trials proved to be safe and effective as a single-oral-dose drug, metrifonate and oxamniquine fell out of favour and out of production. It has been argued that one or both may be useful again if resistance to praziquantel becomes a serious issue, but I doubt that the companies would restart production, since each is a less-than-perfect medication.

Compared to metrifonate and oxamniquine, praziquantel was apparently a wonderdrug, a dream come true. It is safe, results in fewer side-effects, is effective against all schistosome species and, indeed, is now no longer expensive, some 90% cheaper than when it was first marketed.

Alternatives to Praziquantel

Praziquantel (like oxamniquine) is effective against the adult worms but not immature stages. Clearly, we could do with a drug against the immature stages as well. One brief hope emerged (also in the 1980s) with the news that the antimalarial drug artemisinin was effective against immature stages (Fenwick *et al.*, 2006).

To kill two birds with one stone, artemisinin was rapidly trialled in the treatment of *S. japonicum* in China and later in *S. mansoni* and *S. haematobium* in Africa. In the latter two species, artemether and artesunate (different forms of artemisinin) were found to reduce infection by 50% and 25%, respectively, in schoolchildren in highly endemic regions of Cote d'Ivoire.

These results appeared to warrant further investigations, especially in areas that are co-endemic for schistosomiasis and malaria, to see if malaria programmes using artemisinin also opportunistically reduce schistosomiasis. However, a word of warning was issued by the malariologists – 'Because of the danger of inducing resistance by the malaria parasite it is not prudent to target schistosomiasis with any artemisinin derivation' – and so there does not really appear to be any future for the use of artemisinin specifically for schistosomiasis.

One 'notorious' alternative to praziquantel is myrrh. An Egyptian manufacturer produced and marketed it as an effective drug against schistosomiasis – and indeed myrrh has been valued in China, Greece, Egypt and Somalia for centuries as a common analgesic, and even as an antihelminthic and to treat diarrhoea. The Egyptian scientist behind the myrrh product claimed greater than 90% reductions in worm burden in trials in mice infected with *S. mansoni*. However, independent researchers in Egypt, UK and USA were not able to validate these claims, and human trials also failed. The work is now thoroughly discredited.

Finally, the anti-*Fasciola* drug triclabendazole (TCBZ) is another compound which had shown some promising results in mice: its impact on schistosomiasis burden was studied in human populations in Egypt where it is primarily used against *Fasciola* infections (Osman *et al.*, 2011). The study surveyed 6314 people in 15 villages near Alexandria before and after treatment with TCBZ. Prevalence of single infections of schistosomiasis was 15.8%, of fascioliasis alone was 2.2%, and of co-infections was 0.7%. Eight weeks after two doses of TCBZ, the cure rate for fascioliasis was 96% but only 32.7% for schistosomiasis. Those cured had low-intensity infections. The conclusion was that TCBZ was safe but not as effective as praziquantel and could not be recommended for infection with *S. mansoni* alone. However, in areas where both parasitic diseases were present, there was merit in administering TCBZ preceding praziquantel for cases of co-infection. Thus, TCBZ is not considered to be competitive against praziquantel.

Gezira Irrigation Scheme in Sudan

The price of a bottle of local beer

It was on one of my field trips into the Gezira scheme to carry out some molluscide trials that I learned something new about life in the country villages. Because I was going for a couple of weeks I decided I would not take a crate of my favourite local beer with me, because there was no refrigerator in the village hut where I was staying (or to be exact sleeping under the stars). When my driver Meligi suggested I might like a beer on the third night, I must say I was interested. He told me it would cost one Sudanese pound, three times what a beer cost in Khartoum, but then, in a Muslim village in Sudan, I was surprised there was any beer at any price. So off he went with my pound and he came back two hours later with my beer. This was repeated two days later and then two days after that – each time the cost was one pound. Since he was my only company, I was a bit miffed at his long absences, even though he did return with beer. So the next time he asked, I said 'OK, but I will come with you'. This he was not happy with, and he tried vigorously to dissuade me. His final argument was that he had to go to a bad place to get the beer. I could not think what bad place that might be so I pressed him for more details. Finally, he gave in and, sheepishly, said that the beer came from a brothel. I was amazed and said so. 'There is a brothel in the village?' I asked. And he replied, 'Yes'. My curiosity was aroused and I asked him how much the brothel charged for a visit. 'One pound,' he said, and after a pause added, 'but you get a free beer.'

The Rotary Club and hand pumps

The schistosomiasis prevalence in the Gezira irrigation scheme was almost 100%, especially among the settlers living in mud-hut camps on the banks of canals full of snails. These really poor people were immigrants from even poorer places to the west of Sudan and even as far as Nigeria. As 'squatters', they had no facilities provided by the Gezira authorities, nor access to clean, fresh water, nor electricity, and relied on the muddy canal water for all their needs – water that carried both schistosomiasis and cholera.

I was contacted in the late 1970s by Richard Cansdale (elderly readers may remember the name George Cansdale of *Zootime* on TV). Richard

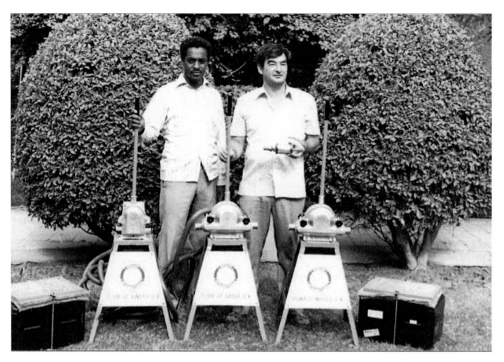

Fig. 4.2. Pumps donated by Rotary.

(George's son) had started a business selling simple hand pumps, which he then marketed through UK Rotary clubs for them to donate to poor countries as part of their international charitable activities. Quite a few UK Rotary clubs bought and shipped pumps to Rotary clubs in the poorest countries in Africa if they could show a need, plus a mechanism for them to be installed. I obtained approval from the Gezira authorities to install pumps in the mud-hut camps of Gezira (each camp usually housing fewer than 50 people).

What we did for these people was to dig a small tunnel through the canal bank below the waterline which allowed canal water to run through. We installed a horizontal roughening filter – basically, a channel full of stones which became a biological filter – and collected the filtered water into a small underground reservoir. The water then passed into a second reservoir through a sand channel and the water in that second reservoir was crystal clear and free of any nasty organisms. The second reservoir was closed but with a hand pump installed, the residents in the small settlements were able to have access to clean water for drinking and cooking.

Every pump was labelled with the name of the donating Rotary club in the UK and photographed to be sent to the donor clubs. Then, whenever I was in the UK, I would visit the donating clubs as a guest speaker and explain, with photographs, just how much their pumps were appreciated and how the provision of clean and filtered canal water would protect the camp dwellers from diarrhoea, cholera and schistosomiasis.

Because of my efforts to provide the pumps to these small settlements, in 1980 I was inducted as a member into the Khartoum Rotary Club, Sudan's only active club. They were a wonderful group, a mixture of different nationalities and occupations. I enjoyed eight years as a member, sitting once a week in an upstairs room in the Nile Hilton, overlooking the junction of the Blue and White Niles where a clear line of the different-coloured water could be seen in the sunlight.

Blue Nile Health Project and an Unhappy ODA Man

In my final years in Sudan (1980–1988) I was assigned by the British government to assist with establishing the Blue Nile Health Project (BNHP) (el Gaddal, 1985), an initiative set up by the government of Sudan. Again, I have George Nelson to thank for that – what a fairy godfather he proved to be (though he had his moments [see 'George, my guest speaker, goes missing', below]).

It was 1980, and George reminded me that my Harvard-Wellcome appointment would cease the following year. He recommended I apply for a post as a principal scientific officer working for Dr John Duncan and the late Peter Haskell at the Centre for Overseas Pest Research (COPR) at Wright's Lane in Kensington. If successful, I would be posted by them back to Sudan as the British government's contribution to the BNHP, which was co-funded by the World Health Organization and the United States Agency for International Development (USAID).

The aim of this project was to control schistosomiasis *and* malaria across the Gezira irrigation scheme, which lies to the south of Khartoum between the two Niles as they converge in Khartoum itself. The area covered 2 million hectares and had 2 million occupants.

The tools to be used for malaria were drugs for treatment of acute malaria combined with prevention using indoor insecticide spraying of huts to kill mosquitoes; and for schistosomiasis, treatment with praziquantel and prevention using some molluscicides in canals near villages. An added schistosomiasis prevention measure was the donation of a concrete latrine slab to every household which dug a pit latrine and built a latrine hut in their compound. I would become Director of Research and Training, working with Dr Asim Daffala under BNHP Director Dr Ahmed Ayoub El Gaddal.

I flew to the UK for the obligatory interview at the Overseas Development Administration (ODA). George and his wife Sheila kindly offered me a bed. On the day of my interview, at Eland House near Victoria Station, I headed in by train while George (I thought) went to his office at LSHTM. I waited to be called in for my interview and, eventually, when my turn came, I was introduced to the panel. The chair was an HR man from ODA (because of the seniority of the post) and the other two were Peter Haskell and an independent consultant – George Nelson! I later learned that George and Peter had developed the job description around me, and so I passed the interview. I owe George such a debt of gratitude. Afterwards, he told me that I nearly was disqualified by the ODA/HR panellist who noted that I had scored 96/100 on their scoring system while the other two candidates had scored only about 45. He concluded that the whole interview was a fix and he was most unhappy. However, as I fitted the qualifications and experience needed, he conceded that I was the man for the job.

I spent the last eight years of my stay in Khartoum working for the BNHP and assisting the local team with research and development of different methods of control, convincing people to take the praziquantel and reducing the prevalence and intensity of infection. It was a most rewarding time.

Getting to Grips with Schistosomiasis Transmission

Before the BNHP was established in 1980, I carried out a number of research projects including studying snail infection rates under natural conditions, and how people polluted the water with excreta.

Ann Allen and I devised a plan to observe water use in the Gezira scheme by sitting on top of a Land Rover with binoculars and counting visits to canals by different people (men, women, boys and girls). We monitored their activities, which ranged from collecting water, defecation, swimming, washing utensils and irrigation. We attempted to measure the risk of each activity and whether some were more involved in transmission than others.

Another research activity involved studying movement of snails in the canals. Once a week, I went to several sites where I believed transmission took place because the water flow was almost stagnant and villagers collected water there. I collected a good number of host snails at each visit, painted their shells with nail varnish and released them back into the canal – a different colour each week. I then counted the number of snails collected that had paint on them from previous weeks. I thought the experiment was going quite well until one day a young boy came along and said, 'Oh, you collect these pretty-coloured snails as well – I have found many of them'. So the results (Fenwick and Amin, 1982) were not quite what I expected.

George, My Guest Speaker, Goes Missing, Thanks to Sudan Airways

George Nelson was involved in a very bizarre incident in 1976 when I was asked to arrange the international guest speaker at the annual Sudan Medical Conference to be held in Khartoum. George agreed to be guest speaker and we sent him a business-class ticket from Heathrow to Khartoum on Sudan Airways. At the time, Sudan Airways had just scrapped their two international planes (Comets), and while they were awaiting the arrival of their new planes (Boeing 707s), they had rented some from British Midland Airways, complete with crews and engineers. The pilots and air hostesses who were part of the package deal certainly livened up the Sudan Club in the evenings.

They were mostly very friendly and every time they came in from London they brought bacon and sausages and other goodies for the Sudan Club members who craved such treats.

I was keen to meet George on his arrival and so was at the airport to meet his 6 am flight on the Tuesday before the conference. The plane did not arrive on time, and I suppose that was no surprise, but by 10 am I was panicking and managed to find a member of Sudan Airways who informed me that the plane had been delayed in Rome due to a technical fault and the pilots being out of work hours. Crew and passengers stayed the night in Rome and the plane was rescheduled to arrive in Khartoum at 6 am on Wednesday. Sadly, it did not arrive, again, and at 10 am on Wednesday I was told that the plane was now on the ground in Athens and that, once again, the pilots were out of hours, so the next expectation was a Thursday-morning arrival. On Thursday morning I went to the airport to be told that the plane had reached Cairo and was expected in Khartoum at 2 pm. At last the plane arrived (60 hours late) and I watched all the passengers disembark, but there was no George Nelson! I waited for the air hostesses to come through. I found someone I recognized and asked her about my Professor. She thought for a minute and said, 'There was an Englishman in business class from London but, come to think of it, I haven't seen him since Athens'. He had disappeared. So, we had no guest speaker at our conference that week, and I was worried and wondered if George was OK. On the Monday morning, a Sudanese gentleman came to my office and asked if I was Dr Alan. When I said I was, he gave me a letter

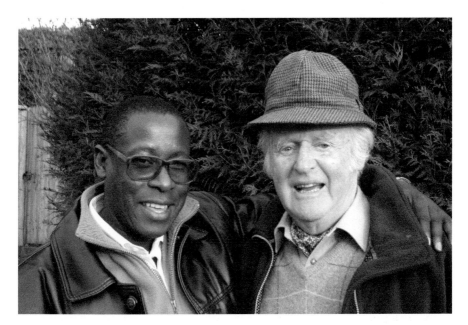

Fig. 4.3. After he retired, Narcis Kabatereine from Uganda and I visited George at his home near Bristol for a fond reunion.

that he said was written in haste by a passenger on the plane on which he had flown in last week from London. It read:

> Dear Alan,
>
> This flight may not get to Khartoum in time for the conference, and actually may never get there at all. I am in Athens, 3 days after leaving London, and have just seen the other Sudan Airways plane on the tarmac on its way to London. I hope you do not mind but I have decided to leave the Khartoum flight and have agreed with Sudan Airways that I can jump on the London plane and go home. I hope that the conference was a success.
>
> Best wishes,
> George.

Extra-curricular Activities in Sudan

I was able to enjoy many extra-curricular activities in Khartoum. I joined the very active amateur dramatic society and volunteered to be the Honorary Secretary of the Sudan Club, where I played squash almost daily and swam in the swimming pool. It was also the setting for my pantomimes (see later). I played cricket every Friday and Saturday on a grass pitch in Khartoum North and I managed a spell as the Chairman of the PTA of the English-speaking primary school where my daughters were enrolled (by now we had three). Our second daughter, Gill, was born in Edinburgh in 1972 and our third daughter, Helen, arrived in 1975, born in Liverpool.

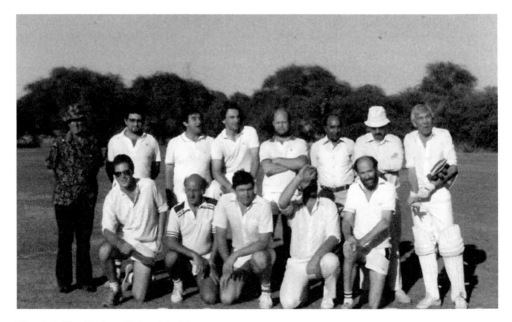

Fig. 4.4. The Sudan Club cricket team.

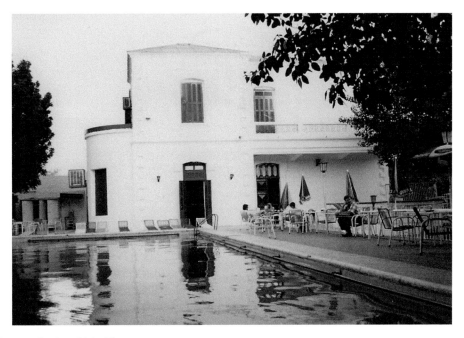

Fig. 4.5. Sudan Club, Khartoum.

The Sudan Club

The Sudan Club was a club in Khartoum exclusively for British passport holders. This was not the British being exclusive; this was the law in Khartoum, and there were many national clubs including Armenian, French, German, Italian and Swiss.

Cricket in Sudan was an experience. There were only 30 players in the country, and we played on a field that had to be flooded on a Sunday to be playable the following weekend (Friday and Saturday). On the plus side, one of our most enthusiastic cricketers was the manager of British Airways in Sudan, and BA would support our annual cricket club ball by flying out a celebrity to play in our match and be guest of honour at the evening event that weekend. BA sent us some top stars of the cricketing world starting with Freddie Trueman, then Majid Khan, Don Wilson, Peter Parfitt, Derek Underwood and Rachel Heyhoe-Flint, among others. I will never forget the time I opened the batting with Majid Khan and we scored 200 for the opening partnership!

The Alan Fenwick pantomimes

And then there was the theatre. Even before Sudan, I had so enjoyed the amateur dramatic experience in Arusha that, on arrival in Khartoum, I

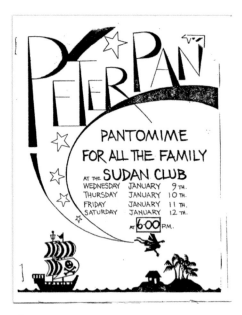

Fig. 4.6. An Alan Fenwick Pantomime programme.

started writing, producing and directing pantomimes in the Sudan Club, staging them every year in early January at the far end of the club's grounds.

The Alan Fenwick Pantomime became an annual event for 16 years and every November I locked myself away and wrote a new, locally inspired, pantomime. December afternoons after work were spent in cast rehearsals until our pantomime was ready to run for four nights in the first week of January, to packed houses.

The English pantomime must be strong in musical content and for that I depended on my wife, Irene. I wrote the words and the songs and Irene, a talented musician, married the words to the music and played the piano accompaniment for every show. I cannot forget the enthusiasm we generated for those productions – enthusiasm by the adult cast members and by every small English child living in Khartoum. Cinderella, Ali Baba, Jack and the Beanstalk, Peter Pan, and Dick Whittington, are but a few of the stories I adapted for the Khartoum stage.

Our three children, Janet, Gill and Helen, all wanted to take part and had to quickly learn lines after returning for the Christmas holidays from their boarding school in the UK. Many of the adults taking part in the shows also had children at boarding school and so they asked if parts could be reserved for their children too. We had so many children in the cast it was a wonder there were enough left to watch the show! Meanwhile, every younger British child who lived in Khartoum sat each afternoon to watch the rehearsals on stage and, of course, they all learned the words off by heart. When it came to the productions we had no need for a prompt because if anyone forgot their lines or even hesitated, the lines were shouted out by these young children sitting on their carpets at the front.

My Farewell Party Piece to Sudan and a Big Surprise

In early 1988, knowing this would be my last year in Sudan, I offered to produce a farewell play on that Sudan Club stage, and we were honoured with the presence of the British Ambassador, John Bevan, in the audience. Speaking to me afterwards, he asked if I could call in at the British Embassy the next day. I turned up at the Embassy and was ushered through security doors and up some stairs to his office, wondering what on earth was going to happen.

After a few niceties, he asked whether I had received a letter from Margaret Thatcher. When I said that I had not, the Ambassador produced a copy of the letter and invited me to read it. It informed me that Margaret Thatcher was going to invite the Queen to appoint me as an Officer of the Order of the British Empire (OBE) and I was asked if I would accept the honour. The Ambassador said that if I agreed (which I did), he would inform No. 10; *but*, I was told to tell no one until the official announcement was made. That was *not* easy!

Ambassador Bevan replied on my behalf and, sure enough, my name was announced as a recipient of the OBE in the Queen's Birthday Honours in June 1988. I am grateful to whoever nominated me – the Khartoum Embassy, perhaps, or my London-based DFID project officer David Turner. I will never know. The Ambassador suggested that we announce the award at a cocktail party at his residence for my friends and colleagues on the evening of the announcement, without the invitation giving anything away. It was a lovely gesture by His Excellency, and much appreciated. Later in 1988, I went to

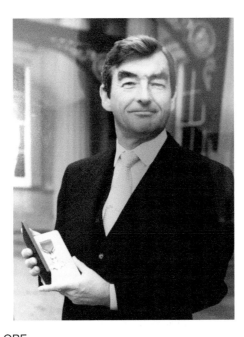

Fig. 4.7. Receiving the OBE.

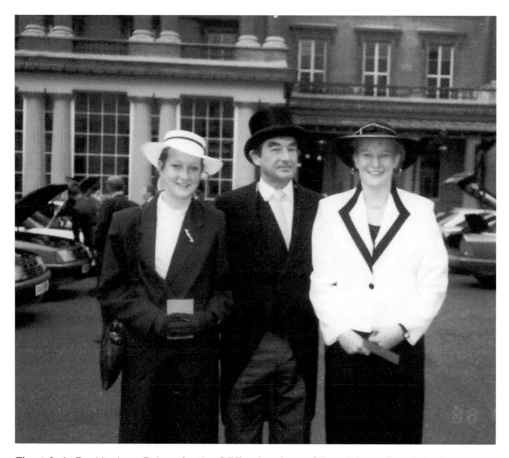

Fig. 4.8. At Buckingham Palace for the OBE – daughters Gill and Janet Fenwick with Alan.

Buckingham Palace to receive the award and could take three guests, which was a bit sad, because I had a wife and three daughters, which meant that my youngest daughter Helen was unable to attend.

At that time, no photographs were allowed at the actual ceremony inside the palace, and so all I have is a photo of myself smirking and holding the medal in the grounds of the palace. Of course, I display those three letters after my name.

My Time in Sudan

In summary, in Sudan I had promoted the careers of several Sudanese colleagues. Together we had rather killed off Frescon as a viable molluscicide and had proved the efficacy of praziquantel. We had improved the lives of millions of people by providing toilets, carrying out indoor spraying against mosquitoes, treating canals to kill snails and reduce transmission where possible, and using praziquantel to treat infected people.

I'd hooked up with Rotary, which became a significant and permanent feature of my life and gained two more daughters and an OBE.

The last eight years there had been difficult, against a backdrop of regular political unrest and the imposition of Sharia law. I had arrived during one period of unrest, back in 1971; when I landed in Khartoum to take up my post I was the only one who got off the plane, and the departure lounge was full of people clamouring to get on it. Apparently, President Numeiri had just nationalized many private businesses and properties, and expatriate businessmen and women were leaving in droves. By 1988, we had survived several coups aimed at removing President Numeiri and there had been extreme shortages of food and petrol from time to time, which made life difficult. One of the worst events during my stay in Sudan was the Black September raid on the Saudi Embassy, which occurred on 1 March 1973, when members of Black September entered the Saudi ambassador's residence during a diplomatic cocktail event and took hostages from among the diplomats who were there.

I had spent five years in Tanzania and 17 years in Sudan, all of which were focused on just one disease, schistosomiasis. What could I do next? What would the future offer me?

5 Assisting the Control of Bilharzia in Egypt, 1988–2002

Death of an Egyptian Singing Star

I was blessed with some more good fortune in 1988 as my time in Sudan was ending. Egypt had been plagued by schistosomiasis since the ancient days of the pharaohs and dynasties and it was where Theodore Bilharz discovered schistosomes as the causal agent of the disease in 1852.

By 1983, despite several control efforts, the prevalence of schistosomiasis in rural Egypt was over 50%, but without an effective drug, snail control appeared to be the best and only method of preventing transmission.

A turning point in the perception of the importance of schistosomiasis came about when Egypt lost one of its most famous singers, Abdel Halim Hafez, in 1977, to complications of the disease in the liver due to a heavy infection of *Schistosoma mansoni*. The country went into mourning, and bilharzia became a household name and an infection everyone feared.

The government was primed to take on the challenge of controlling schistosomiasis, and luck played a part in determining my joining that challenge. In September 1978, Egypt's president, Anwar Sadat, and Israel's prime minister, Menachem Begin, both attended a conference at Camp David, the US president's country retreat in Maryland. The president of the USA, Jimmy Carter, brokered a peace agreement with these two leaders, launching a period of fragile peace between their nations. Sadly, this peace deal cost President Sadat his life because he was assassinated in October 1981 by fundamentalist dissidents.

In return for the peace agreement, the USA funded a number of projects to improve the economic situation in Egypt. These included roads, education, telecommunications and housing, but for health, the Egyptians asked for assistance to control bilharzia. The USA agreed and their USAID office in Cairo was appointed to arrange for the neatly named Schistosomiasis Research Project (SRP) to be designed and implemented by Medical Services Corporation International (MSCI), a 'contractor' based in Arlington, Virginia.

MSCI brought in a high-powered team chaired by one Dr F. DeWolfe Miller, a professor of epidemiology at Hawaii University. His team read like a *Who's Who* of USA schistosomiasis experts at the time – Dan Colley, Phil LoVerde, Mike Phillips, Clive Shiff, Barnett Cline and Robert (Bob) Lennox.

© Fenwick, Norris and McCall 2022. *A Tale of a Man, a Worm and a Snail: The Schistosomiasis Control Initiative* (A. Fenwick *et al.*)
DOI: 10.1079/9781786392558.0005

When the project document was completed, MSCI was invited by USAID to implement the first nine months of the SRP as 'interim contractor', which they accepted once it was confirmed that this would not preclude them from bidding to manage the full ten-year project.

They needed a Chief of Party, and Bob Lennox, their chief scientific advisor and right-hand man to the CEO, without ever having met me, decided that I was the person to do the job. He tracked me down by calling my mother in Liverpool – I never did find out how he managed to reach her – and she told him I would be at the Sudan Club at 4.30 pm every day, as I always was after work, either swimming or playing squash. No one had a private telephone in their home in Khartoum in those days and mobile phones, as we know them today, were not available. Somehow, Bob found the telephone number of the Sudan Club and made the call to try to reach me. The manager was totally surprised to receive a call from the USA; 'That's a first,' he said, but he sent a runner to drag me out of the squash court. Bob asked me whether I would take the job as interim Chief of Party, living in Cairo, with the job of (a) setting up the terms of reference of the SRP; and (b) preparing the bid for the MSCI to manage the project for ten years with me as Chief of Party. Obviously, I agreed.

I think in 17 years in Sudan I received less than ten international calls, so getting this one was rather special. All credit to Bob Lennox for his perseverance. In the time I was in Sudan I hardly made an international phone call home because this meant a visit to the Grand Hotel, 'tipping' the telephone operator to make the call, waiting in a queue for at least an hour, all for a three-minute chat.

SRP Established in Cairo, 1988

The SRP in Egypt was established in 1988 in the Ministry of Health facility at VACSERA (a research centre in Mohandeseen, Cairo), and I went there to set up the project with no guarantee that I could stay the full ten years. Because of the uncertainty, I did not rent an apartment but lived alone in the Nile Hilton Hotel for the first nine months, pessimistically expecting to have to leave SRP at the end of that time. Naturally, living alone, I had more 'off-duty' time than normal. What I needed to fill it was to join the Gezira Club on Zamalek Island, just across the Nile from the hotel, where I could play squash and golf. Joining the Gezira Club was a bit expensive, but after a particularly successful evening at the hotel's casino, when my roulette numbers (16 and 17) came up four times in succession, I had enough to pay for six months' membership.

The bid I prepared with colleagues on behalf of MSCI in those nine months duly won and I was confirmed as Chief of Party. This meant a ten-year stay in Egypt and so I had to find a flat. I found No. 4, Hassan Asim Street, Zamalek. I did wonder why I was chosen for the job (leaving aside any issues over qualifications) and concluded that living and working in the Middle East for ten years was not such an attractive proposition for career-minded (and possibly safety-conscious) Americans – thus leaving the way open for me.

This is when I was joined by Margie Wright as my partner. I had first met Margie, an entomologist from Zimbabwe based in the UK, in 1987 when she was researching crop pests in Sudan. I had been asked to introduce her to the Sudan Club and we kept in touch when she returned to the UK in 1988. She joined me in Cairo in 1989 and we were married in Dumfries, Scotland, in 1993 after the divorce from Irene was finalized.

I eagerly took on the management of the SRP from 1988 through to 1998; an operational research project with a $40 million budget. As Chief of Party, I was responsible for the day-to-day running, procurement, scientific over-sight and management of all the activities of 100 Egyptian and US research scientists. During my time in control, I would negotiate about 50 grants, plan the training of staff and manage the fundamental mechanics of having money and equipment in place to keep the project ticking over on the ground, all the while having to follow the US government's strict procurement policy of buying US products where possible. The phrase 'America First' comes to mind (I wonder why?).

World Bank Offers Additional $40 Million Support for Control

More good fortune was to follow. The SRP launch and USAID's donation for research coincided with the World Bank agreeing another US$40 million support for control measures in Egypt and this included money to purchase the drug praziquantel so that it could be made available, free of charge, to rural Egyptians through the Ministry of Health. With this extra funding, the ministry started a control campaign – the World Bank Control Project – based on diagnosis and treatment using the drug. (Previous campaigns had focused on reducing transmission by killing snails.) The permanent under-secretary responsible for schistosomiasis control was Dr Taha El Khoby, and the Egyptian minister of health made the decision to make him responsible for both the research (the SRP) and the control programmes. For the next ten years my office was next to Dr Taha's and we collaborated closely together to conduct research into schistosomiasis and run a national control programme.

National TV Campaign to Raise Awareness

The control campaign was supported by a series of very clever advertise-ments, made locally and shown regularly on Egyptian TV, urging people to go to be tested and treated if infected. The recurring message was 'Now we have pills not injections like before' and 'Turn your back to the canal'. The idea of turning your back to the canal was to prevent people urinating into the water, but it became the source of great amusement and ridicule in Egypt. These adverts were a constant source of conversation and people were openly talking about bilharzia.

Dr Taha and I promised the World Bank that with their funding we would reduce the prevalence of infection, the number of people with heavy infections (intensity of infection) and the morbidity of schistosomiasis by regular annual treatment of children and infected adults with praziquantel. The target was that schistosomiasis would no longer be considered a public health problem. In practice, that meant no more deaths from either bladder cancer or haematemesis (bleeding from oesophageal varices).

Dr Taha El Khoby was a most astute but gentle man for whom I developed great respect and a close friendship. His deputy, Dr Nabil Galal, led the research side of the project to great effect and we hired a local training expert, Madam Olfat, to be responsible for the training plans. Perhaps the most notorious staff member was my personal assistant, Miss Siham Omer El Kafafi, who can only be described as the project's dynamo. Siham was a joy to have in the office and she managed me and the project very efficiently.

Building a Team and Enhancing My Education

The SRP became a huge part of my life and, frankly, it was the SRP and the many people that I worked with during my 14 years in Egypt that set me up for establishing the SCI in 2002.

As Chief of Party, I was based in Cairo but some of my MSCI staff members were home-based in Arlington, Virginia. They included Bob Lennox, as Deputy Director of MSCI, Home Office Manager Dr Pat Carney and Grants Manager Richard Joseph. We worked very closely together, with both Pat and Richard making frequent visits to Egypt.

Working with USAID

Working with USAID was a real revelation because they are so 'in your face' with very close involvement and supervision, not to mention the intense financial scrutiny. We were audited regularly to ensure we had followed the 'Buy America' rule as far as possible. My first USAID project officer was Dr Sharif Arif, an Egyptian scientist who later transferred to USAID headquarters in Washington.

By the end of the ten-year programme, the project officer to whom I reported was Dr Rick Rhoda, who was a really supportive supervisor and a keen golfer. We could be found regularly, at dawn, playing nine holes at the Gezira Club before work. At the other end of the scale was Linda Lou Kelly, who was the most frustrating supervisor I have ever had the misfortune to work with. Hard as I tried, I just could not engage with her, and all our American investigators and members of our scientific board found her difficult to interact with on a friendship or professional basis. At the more senior level, I was fortunately able to bounce my problems off Mellen Tanamly and, latterly, Duncan Miller. Duncan and his English wife Patricia ended up living opposite us in Mansour Mohamad Street in Zamalek and so we saw a lot of them socially as well as professionally.

In Cairo, I managed to engage with Egyptians, expatriates and visitors through several different routes, and all were very helpful to me, professionally and socially. These included the USAID Funding Circle, the British Businessman's Association, the Gezira Club and then the Rotary.

As for Rotary, it reached me that several local and expatriate businessmen were getting together to start an English-language Rotary Club, the first English-language club in Egypt. I expressed an interest, and in 1990 I became a founder member of the Cairo Cosmopolitan Rotary Club with, maybe, 15 Egyptians and 15 expatriates from various countries. Our Monday breakfast meetings really were wonderful and a great way to meet new people since there was quite a turnover of expatriates. I became President of the Club in 1994 and had a successful year except for one blip – I introduced Cheryl Wynne-Eyton into the club, the first-ever lady Rotarian in Egypt; this was not well received by some members and a few Egyptians left to join a male-only club. However, I think it was their loss because Cheryl proved to be an excellent Rotarian and the Cosmopolitan Club is now a truly mixed-gender club.

Our Circle of Friends Opens Up

The year after establishing the SRP in Egypt, when I was joined by Margie Wright (now my wife of over 25 years), my life changed from being alone in a hotel room in Zamalek to entertaining many schistosomiasis experts at our home and enjoying a most wonderful life of work and social events.

Our neighbours across the road in Zamalek included Andy and Julia Henderson and their children Emma and Amelia. They became lifelong friends and we visited them on a subsequent posting to South Africa and then at their home in Salisbury when they retired from the Foreign Office. Indeed, generally, in all my postings we have gained lifelong friends and colleagues.

When I partnered with Margie, a host of friends from her past became our friends, but none more closely than John and Di Donaldson who had been at Rhodes University with Margie in the late 1970s in Grahamstown, South Africa. We have had some great meetings with the Donaldsons over the years in Cape Town where they live, or meeting up with mutual friends in UK and Spain. Only once did our work cause our paths to cross, since John is a specialist in animal and plant ecology. By chance, in Nairobi, John and I were at different meetings; his was on ecology of African animals whilst mine was to meet with African Ministry of Health officials reporting on NTD progress.

That gave Margie and Di the chance to spend some great times together, which gave rise to some wonderful additions to our photograph collection, including ones at the giraffe sanctuary in Nairobi, where visitors stand on a

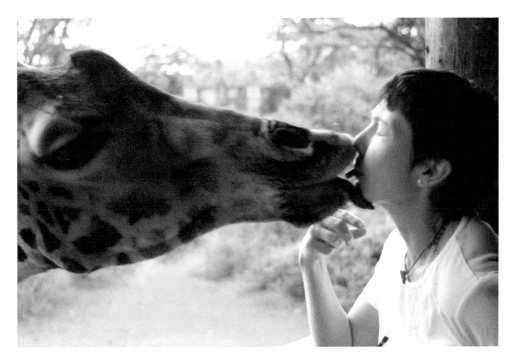

Fig. 5.1. Margie feeds a giraffe at a sanctuary in Nairobi.

wooden platform to feed giraffes with food pellets. Of course, Margie and Di had to be different, and they put the pellets between their lips so the giraffe had to come close and almost kiss them to retrieve the pellets!

Getting Around in Cairo

Those who have visited Cairo will know how bad the traffic is and so it was essential that I had not only a project vehicle but that Margie and I also had a private car. With parking in Cairo a massive problem, this meant we needed drivers for each vehicle, to drop us off, wait in the car somewhere nearby and then pick us up after our meeting, shopping, meal, or whatever else we might be doing. The project driver employed by the Ministry of Health was Refat Younan, who stayed with me for all of 13 years; and for the private car (a Mercedes) we owned we had an elderly gentleman called Edward, who was such a wonderful person and took great care of us *and* the car.

Margie and the 'Befrienders'

While I was working with Dr Taha, Margie was not standing idly by; she and her friend Dr Lillian Craig Harris established Befrienders Cairo (a branch of

the Samaritans, which outside the UK is known as Befrienders International).
I became their fundraiser.

Lillian was the wife of Alan Goulty, who was then deputy head of
the British Embassy in Cairo. I had actually known Alan from his time in
Sudan where he was famous for winning the Sudan Open tennis tourna-
ment one year against some strong Sudanese players. The Goultys and
the Fenwicks became close and we holidayed together not only in Egypt
but also, later, in Uganda. After Alan and Lillian retired, they moved to
Washington, DC, and as I was a frequent visitor to DC by that time (as you
will discover), every time I went there I called them and either dined with
them on one of my nights there or they came to my hotel and had breakfast
or dinner with me. Then, on one of my shorter visits, I neglected to call. I
thought, 'Never mind, they will not know I was there'. I went to fly back
to London and got on a British Airways Boeing 777 and was upgraded
to business class. I took my seat and the man who had the window seat
arrived, and as I got up to let him in I realized it was Alan Goulty. Another
lesson learned!

Once she had her work visa, Margie worked as a technical assistant with
Dr Moamena Kamel, a clinical pathologist who owned a string of clinical
and diagnostic laboratories. (Dr Moamena was also one of the SRP Egyptian
Project Investigators (PI) and her US collaborator on diagnostics was Dr
F. DeWolfe Miller.) But this didn't stop her Befriender activities, which
included recruiting volunteers. One who became famous among visiting
friends and scientists was a gemologist named Sharif Begermi. He thought
he might become a volunteer, but, on learning more about the organization,
he decided instead to become a donor, donating jewellery pieces for auctions
or raffles at fundraising events. Margie would take any US or British wives
to his Cairo showrooms in Opera Square.

In the last few years in Cairo, Margie even found time to start a small
business helping settle expatriates into the city. On our return to the UK,
she continued to work with the Samaritans. She eventually retrained as a
psychotherapist and now runs a successful practice where we live.

Entertaining Visitors, and Adventures in Egypt

Some special people and events

One of our visitors, a US collaborating scientist called Dr Michael Phillips,
turned out to be slightly naïve on his first visit. He had agreed to host a
young Egyptian from the SRP as a PhD student at his university in the USA,
and when Mike was due to come to Egypt the young man asked him to bring
over a present for his family. Without questioning the student, Mike arrived
at Cairo airport with rather a lot of luggage and was searched at customs.
The several video players and other electrical goods in the parcel were all
confiscated by the customs officers and Mike was lucky to escape arrest on
charges of smuggling.

the hills. I sat tight and the owner had to run up the path to stop my disappearing. I should point out that several donkeys were used in the filming. As we started the second run-through we noticed the donkey had become a bit excited, not only braying loudly but also displaying an erection for all to see! Cold water was needed before the second shoot could be completed!

The exciting part of the filming covered Howard Carter entering the tomb and finding all the wonders that were there. For this we returned to Cairo and received permission to film Carter's entrance into a replica of Tutankhamen's tomb, which had been built on the banks of the Nile in an Egyptian 'historical replica' site owned by a Rotarian friend of mine Dr Abdel Salam Ragab. It was quite a learning curve, both to learn more about the contents of the tomb but also the detail that goes into making a film, and just how much film they take compared to how little of it they use.

After this short interlude I had to get back to the control of schistosomiasis in Egypt!

Egypt Virtually Eliminates Schistosomiasis, 1990–2002

Despite being considerably wealthier in terms of GDP than the sub-Saharan African countries that were to become the focus for the later SCI project, Egypt shares some distinct parallels with them in terms of disease settings. Most notably, the disadvantaged in rural Egypt depend on agriculture for their living, as do most of the populations in Burkina Faso, Mali, Niger, Tanzania, Uganda or Zambia (the countries supported by the SCI). Likewise, there is the same need for advocacy at every level from ministries of health and education through to schoolchildren. These rural agricultural populations usually must survive on less than $2 a day, which is hard enough at the best of times, but when someone in the family is ill or new clothes are needed, the effect is devastating.

The main difference with sub-Saharan African countries is that in Egypt there were more medical facilities available to serve the poor people, and many more doctors per head of population. It also developed very quickly in the 1990s with USAID support, and two aspects of their support were supplying electricity and clean water to rural villages.

Egypt Makes Cheap Praziquantel with EIPICO

Egypt also had a manufacturing base, and because of the World Bank funding (and USAID support), an Egyptian pharmaceutical company (EIPICO) entered an agreement with Shin Poong (a Korean-based pharmaceutical company) who were making cheap, high-quality praziquantel (see Chapter 7). With this arrangement, EIPICO won the tender to supply the Egyptian Ministry of Health with praziquantel for their World Bank-funded MDA programme to treat all the children in endemic areas.

This became pivotal in persuading the Egyptian government to allocate further resources to schistosomiasis, remembering the knowledge about schistosomiasis amongst the population was already high following the death of Abdel Halim Hafez. In sub-Saharan countries, different ministries fought fiercely over limited funds, and schistosomiasis was not as high a priority as it was in Egypt. Few governments would readily divert already limited health sector money away from HIV or malaria to something with a low profile. In contrast, by 1988 Egypt was free of malaria, and HIV was quite rare, so that removed the major competitors for health sector resources.

The plan we developed for the SRP, and approved by USAID, had two main objectives: to provide the Egyptian government with better tools to manage the disease; and to build capacity amongst Egyptian scientists to conduct biomedical research. The emphasis of the SRP was therefore infinitely more on the research aspect of schistosomiasis, leaving the Ministry of Health staff to place their major emphasis on implementation using World Bank resources.

Research Proposals – the Rules Governing the SRP

Once the SRP Secretariat was established within the VACSERA compound in Mohandiseen, the SRP invited several established Egyptian investigators to submit proposals for research into five aspects of schistosomiasis (epidemiology, snail control, immunology, chemotherapy and vaccine development). Each proposal was considered only if there was an internationally renowned US collaborator who was willing to visit Egypt maybe twice a year to participate in the research. Through this mechanism, I was able to recruit some well-qualified Egyptian principal investigators and some expert US scientists, with whom we shared some great experiences over ten years (1988–1998). These scientists came together every two years when I organized an international conference on schistosomiasis in Cairo (and once in Sharm El-Sheikh). We also met up annually at the ASTMH meetings, which, like many scientific conferences, change venues each time, and in this case moved around the cities of the USA. Conferences are an important part of capacity building in science, advancing science and careers. They are where one can hear about other people's research, compare notes, make friendships and set up collaborations; and look for the next opportunity for funding, training or a research position.

After ten years of the World Bank-funded control project, the Ministry of Health had conclusively demonstrated that schistosomiasis could be effectively controlled at the national level using praziquantel to treat infected populations[1] on an annual basis (so called 'morbidity control'). The data showed that the prevalence of schistosomiasis outside of Cairo was reduced from about 25% in 1988 to less than 2% in 2004 (Figure 5.6).

Meanwhile, among the products of the SRP research (El Khoby *et al.*, 1998) funded by USAID were: a formulation of praziquantel suitable for very young children; an established resistance monitoring and reporting centre; results from a large epidemiological study to measure the scale of

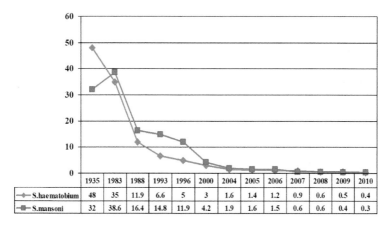

	1935	1983	1988	1993	1996	2000	2004	2005	2006	2007	2008	2009	2010
S.haematobium	48	35	11.9	6.6	5	3	1.6	1.4	1.2	0.9	0.6	0.5	0.4
S.mansoni	32	38.6	16.4	14.8	11.9	4.2	1.9	1.6	1.5	0.6	0.6	0.4	0.3

Fig. 5.6. The successful control of schistosomiasis in Egypt (Fenwick, 2017).

disease across the country; health education materials for TV; novel snail control measures (such as slow-release formulation of niclosamide); dipstick diagnostic tests which changed colour in a urine sample taken from an infected person; and experience of using ultrasound as a diagnostic tool to uncover liver damage. SRP had also assisted WHO in its attempts to develop a vaccine against schistosomiasis.

At the governmental level, the Ministry of Health now had an effective strategy for the control of schistosomiasis and a geographical information system (GIS) for monitoring disease distribution; and the country found itself with a fully trained and equipped scientific community capable of bio-medical research and almost 100 peer-reviewed published scientific papers to their names (Schistosomiasis Research Project, 2000). Most importantly, because of the parallel World Bank control project, rural Egypt now had a population of children with a future free of the terrible consequences of schistosomiasis (no blood in the urine, no ascites and no early death from vomiting blood or cancer of the bladder).

As a direct result of these two projects, today, schistosomiasis is no longer a public health problem in Egypt, and bladder cancer – once the most common cancer of all in the 1960s – is now very rare indeed.

Success in Egypt – a Springboard to Future Ambition

In terms of what was to follow, the SRP and the World Bank control project served as excellent springboards from which to tackle schistosomiasis in sub-Saharan Africa. In 2002, when I left Egypt, I could boast a track record of managing successful research and implementation in Egypt, which I would continue to expand when I started the SCI. I also had what I believed were achievable ambitions of control in all of sub-Saharan Africa. I felt confident that the Egyptian success would attract funding from the wealthy foundations, bilateral government donors and high-net-worth individual donors if we could reach them and promise a similar prevalence reduction as had been achieved in Egypt.

However, I had to demonstrate management and business skills as much as my scientific and research experience to make the future SCI a success. Having sold Egypt as living proof that a large-scale national control programme could work, SCI would need to present a plan to convince government ministers in recipient countries for whom the control of neglected tropical diseases was not a priority in 2002. Our plans had to show clearly that, at minimal cost to the country, any funding we raised for their schistosomiasis programme ended up supporting delivery of medications in rural areas and praziquantel pills arriving in the right mouths.

The WHO World Health Assembly Commits Ministers of Health in Africa to Schistosomiasis Control

In May 2001, before I left Egypt, the 54th World Health Assembly passed a resolution supported by the African ministers of health, affirming their commitment to promoting schistosomiasis control based on a series of core strategies which focused on morbidity control rather than transmission control.[2] This resolution, which was promoted by Morocco, stated that 'all member states where these infections are endemic should provide regular treatment for schistosomiasis and intestinal helminths (also known as soil-transmitted helminths or STH) to at least 75% of all school-aged children in highly endemic areas by the year 2010'. Despite this resolution, for the next five years SCI was the only external driving force and external financial support for any treatments being delivered in sub-Saharan Africa.

But, in 2000, SCI did not exist; all that did exist was the ambition to put praziquantel to good use and to make it accessible to the 200 million infected people in Africa. SCI began from a baseline where not a single country in sub-Saharan Africa had an effective schistosomiasis control programme in their ministry of health.

The SCI, as you will see, is a story of something developed out of nothing, achieved by the collaboration, co-operation and dedication of teams of people from many walks of life; by utilizing the donations of medicines from pharmaceutical companies on an unprecedented scale; with financial donations from governments, individuals and foundations; and the efforts of all the African governments to deliver these medicines to their rural populations.

Notes

[1] Definition of 'infected populations': populations in which there were enough infected individuals to merit mass drug administration delivered annually.
[2] Morbidity control relies on mass drug administration to people; transmission control relies on snail control, usually through molluscides.

6 An Ambitious Programme for Africa (from 2002)

When I left Egypt my ambition had reached the point of the delivery of medicine to everyone in Africa who needed it to fight schistosomiasis – two-thirds of all those on the continent – and where possible to eliminate the transmission of the disease.

Having started on a relatively small but expanding scale, I had shown in Tanzania what needed to be done, and subsequently what could be done on a larger scale in Sudan and then on a national level in Egypt.

From 2002 to 2020, successful control of schistosomiasis was demonstrated through the efforts of SCI supporting local ministries of health and education to treat their school-aged children with the widespread use of praziquantel.

Before the advent of SCI, African governments failed to proactively accept or even recognize that this parasitic disease was a significant public health issue in need of attention, because of its apparently low morbidity. It was truly a neglected tropical disease. In fairness, another factor was that the price of praziquantel was, initially, too high for governments with a small health budget to buy the drug in sufficient quantities to treat all those infected (over 200 million in Africa) on an annual basis. This constraint was only removed or reduced when the price did drop significantly to a level reasonable for mass use, thanks to Shin Poong.

Timing was everything, and my leaving Egypt having completed a 14-year term implementing a most successful national control programme coincided with a change in the global philosophy of philanthropy as well as with relatively cheap praziquantel.

SCI – The Plan – It Happened One Night

Many large-scale successful programmes initially rely on one event or one person's focused interest to ignite enthusiasm and call potential partners to action. In the case of the SCI, I was lucky. I was in the right place at the right time and fortunate enough to have made friends in the right places. I was a parasitologist, fascinated for 40 years by the worms in Africa but horrified by the damage they had done to so many people helpless to resist them.

The initial plan was developed and drafted in 1999 in Brazil. Margie and I had taken the opportunity to visit friends in Brasilia, and then attend the schistosomiasis conference hosted biannually in Brazil (in 1999 it was in Rio de Janeiro).

I awoke one night in Rio, waking up Margie, too, with the overpowering idea that the millions of school-aged children in Africa deserved to be offered a treatment against schistosomiasis. My hypothesis was that an annual school-based programme in endemic areas would immediately improve their quality of life and protect them from serious disease in later life.

Margie and I would reach out to the Bill and Melinda Gates Foundation. The foundation had been launched just two years previously and was destined to be the new source of serious funding for good causes. Already they had funded GAVI (Global Access to Vaccine Initiative or the Vaccine Alliance for short) to deliver vaccines cheaply to children in poor countries.

But would Mr Gates consider schistosomiasis control as a worthwhile cause? I definitely had the enthusiasm for my cause but did I possess the charisma to sell my belief to others, and especially to Mr Gates? At the time, the foundation seemed the only possible source for the level of funding I would need. So I set out, in 2000, on a course to persuade the foundation to let me try to save at least one generation of children in rural Africa from the debilitating effects of a worm-borne disease with praziquantel (de-worming with albendazole was a later addition to the plan).

How could I get through the foundation's door and reach someone in authority? Luck was on my side, not just one stroke of luck but a series of interlocking events which opened that door.

A Series of Fortunate Events

It all started some 30 years earlier. In 1972, I met the famous clinician Dr Joe Cook, who had been the doctor on the 1960s St Lucia Schistosomiasis Research and Control Project when he was on a visit to Sudan. When he left St Lucia he became the International Health Project Officer for the Edna McConnell Clark Foundation, based in New York and funded by the owner of Avon Cosmetics. The foundation spent its money on four categories of need, and one of those categories was international health. Joe was employed as director of their international programmes and his brief was to fund schistosomiasis research projects including a search for a vaccine.

By 1998, I had been in Egypt for ten years managing USAID's funds as Chief of Party to the Schistosomiasis Research Project. By 2000, Joe and I had worked together on several occasions, and met not only in Sudan, Egypt and St Lucia but also at many of the annual conferences of the American Society of Tropical Medicine and Hygiene. We had become friends as well as colleagues.

When USAID closed the SRP in 1998, I was set for an early retirement. However, USAID decided that one section of the SRP should continue for another four years in the hope that a vaccine might be successfully developed.

My future in Egypt, however, looked as if it was stalling because of USAID's bureaucracy and their wish to hire a new contractor. They decided to invite PATH, a Seattle-based NGO with a 'centrally funded USAID programme', which meant that they could mobilize funding quickly to keep the momentum of the vaccine studies going. PATH was reluctant to accept the task of managing this project because of their base in Seattle, which was some distance from Egypt, and they had no expertise on schistosomiasis, nor of Egypt, on their staff. Joe Cook knew Dr Gordon Perkin, the CEO of PATH, well and so he introduced me to him with the suggestion that I was what PATH needed. Because of that introduction I was invited to Seattle for an interview and was quickly employed by PATH using their USAID funding to take the ongoing schistosomiasis vaccine development project through to completion. I was posted back to Egypt, and thanks to Joe and Gordon I stayed another four years in Cairo funded by USAID through PATH. I guess I did a good-enough job to have impressed Dr Perkin because of what happened later.

Developing a vaccine against schistosomiasis was never going to be easy back then – and, in fact, it is probably not much nearer success today. USAID decided to abandon their efforts in 2002. With the project apparently going to fail for lack of funds (though eventually it failed due to scientific difficulties), it was suggested that I approach the Bill and Melinda Gates Foundation who might be interested in supplying the funding needed to see the project through.

I set about preparing a proposal bringing in all the vaccinologists I could rustle up – Alan Wilson (York), Don Harn (Harvard), Miriam Tendler (FioCruz), Ed Pearce (New York) to name a few, all of whom had been involved with vaccine development with Egyptian colleagues at SRP. Our proposal for the Schistosomiasis Vaccine Project was submitted to the foundation early in 1999. But just as there were many people who supported the investment to find a vaccine against schistosomiasis, there were others who passionately opposed such an investment as a waste of money – and none more so than Jim Bennett, a long-time colleague of mine from Sudan days. The views of the anti-vaccine lobby reached the ears of the decision makers in the foundation and our proposal was summarily rejected at the first read-through, deemed unfundable and not value for money. The letter I received said that the Gates Foundation would never support research and development of a vaccine against schistosomiasis. This seemed to be the end of my fundraising initiative.

And so to the biannual Brazil schistosomiasis conference and that special night at 3 am when Margie woke and found me tapping away on my computer. I defended my actions by saying I had the answer to the control of schistosomiasis; not a vaccine but a 'morbidity vaccine', praziquantel. Had we not successfully used this medicine in Egypt, delivering over 70 million treatments with virtually no side-effects and therefore was it not proven to be safe and effective?

Because of using praziquantel over a ten-year period, funded by the World Bank, the prevalence of schistosomiasis in Egypt had fallen to approximately 2% from 20% in 1988. Surely, I thought, Bill Gates would be impressed by these results and see that providing treatment to the children in rural sub-Saharan Africa would be a real value-for-money investment for his foundation. Surely this was a project which would meet the foundation's worthy objectives.

Furthermore, I was inspired by the reduced price of praziquantel: we would have very little trouble in selling the idea of school-based schisto-somiasis control programmes to ministers of health quoting 50 cents per child per year for a safe and effective treatment. I recruited Margie to the idea, planning that, if successful, we could perhaps run it from Zimbabwe from whence she came. So I was encouraged to continue, and prepared my concept note for proof of principle. I hypothesized that ministries of health in Africa would embrace the idea of treating children, providing we made the medicines and funding available, and I submitted it to the foundation. When it arrived at the Gates Foundation it was given to their new Chief Scientific Programme Officer to review – none other than Dr Gordon Perkin who had just retired as CEO of PATH to take up the position as Bill Gates' Scientific Advisor.

My concept note was read and considered, and I think it was because of my previous successful work with PATH in Egypt that I was invited to make a case in Seattle. However, the message from the foundation was

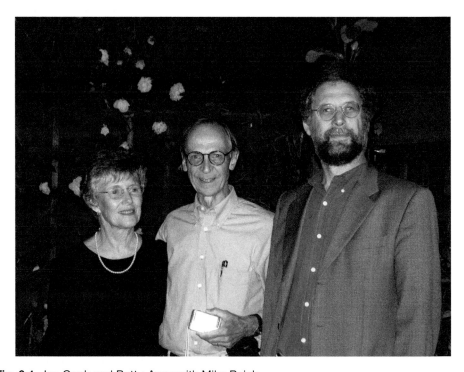

Fig. 6.1. Joe Cook and Betty-Anne with Mike Reich.

that they would not fund me working from Egypt or Zimbabwe but would only give a grant to a recognized academic institution in the USA or UK. I needed an ally in a suitable institution, someone respected and experienced to help me put it across. Again, Dr Joe Cook came to my rescue; he introduced me to Professor Michael Reich from the Harvard School of Public Health, and on Joe's recommendation, Michael agreed to help me. We worked together on an expanded document and shortly afterwards we were invited to Seattle to present the project and make our case to the foundation.

We were grilled by the senior policy staff – Patti Stonesifer and Sylvia Matthews. Also present was Sally Stansfield who later became our first project officer. Those three gave us a hard time with their incisive cross-questioning, but when our time was up, we seemed to have made a positive impression.

Travelling Across Africa to Develop Our Proposal

We were then invited to prepare a slightly different (but still very short) pre-proposal which would request funds for me to spend a year paying visits to African countries and draw up plans to provide medication to millions of rural people in several African countries. The 'exploratory' grant of $750,000 Michael and I requested was approved and paid to the Harvard School of Public Health and for the next six months I travelled the length and breadth of Africa sending data back to Michael so we could prepare a full implementation proposal. As the extent of the need became obvious, I started dreaming. My first thought had been to ask the foundation for $1 million – a huge grant in those days – but soon that became insufficient. Maybe $10 million, or $20 million, or $40 million. And then I thought, with $100 million I could support full coverage of Africa.

Within six months I had visited Kenya, Malawi, Tanzania, Uganda and Zambia in East Africa, and Mali, Burkina Faso, Cameroon and Niger in West Africa, and planned to visit several others. I had talked to the ministers of health where I could reach them, and other senior staff members where I could not. Every government official agreed they needed schistosomiasis treatments, but none of them had money, de-worming drugs, logistical support or the necessary human resources to run a national programme. However, remarkably, in every country there was a schistosomiasis control officer. Usually, he or she had been trained in either the Danish Bilharzia Laboratory or the London School of Hygiene and Tropical Medicine. They each had one thing in common: in every country the schistosomiasis or bilharzia control officer was a sad figure sitting in an office without the tools to do the job.

I met them all: Narcis Kabatereine in Uganda, Samuel Jemu in Malawi, James Mwansa in Zambia, Moussa Sacko and Mamadou Traore in Mali, Amadou Garba in Niger, Ursuline Nyandindi in Tanzania, Seydou Touré in Burkina Faso, Louis Albert Tchuem-Tchuente in Cameroon, Eric Muchiri in Kenya – all well trained to PhD level, all keen and willing to control

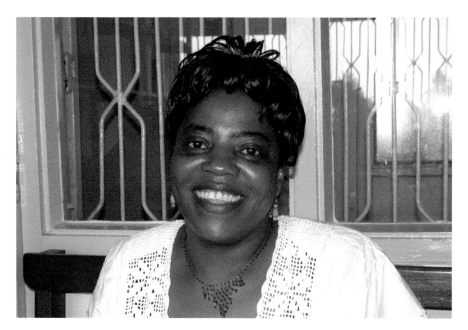

Fig. 6.2. Ursuline Nyandindi.

schistosomiasis in their country, and each one frustrated by the lack of resources and lack of support from within their ministry.

The Winning Proposal

So as the year went by the proposal was taking shape, thanks to Michael Reich and two of his graduate students Scott Gordon and Beatrice Bezmalinovic. But several months before it was ready, Sally Stansfield phoned and asked for the proposal. I was confused and not a little worried – I wasn't ready – I thought I had been given a year. Would I lose everything? 'Well,' she said, 'at least tell me how much will you ask for; we need to budget, and we are preparing our budget for next year'.

'OK, $50 million please,' I heard myself say.

End of telephone call – end of a dream? But eventually the decision came back. 'Sorry, the budget committee considered your verbal proposal and $50 million will not be forthcoming – can you manage with $34 million, and if so, please prepare a proposal of up to ten pages as soon as possible.'

When I calmed down I realized the trouble I was in; to get that $34 million, Michael, Scott, Beatrice and I had to present a perfect proposal – and Michael *is* a perfectionist. However, another realization hit me: if I was successful, I could do so much with $34 million, but not everything – some of those countries I had visited would have to be left out.

The next three months were spent with Michael Reich who is a wizard, and with Scott and Beatrice to assist, preparing the proposal. And what a proposal-writing process it was; I learned so much. My fourth iteration would have been rejected I am now sure, but the fifteenth draft eventually was submitted – and many hours of discussion and deep thought and rewriting went into reaching that stage. If I never thanked them enough then, let me do so now. I am where I am today because of them.

The proposal was submitted early in 2000, but it was not approved immediately. Sally called me and said that she wanted to use our proposal to test out a new foundation review mechanism; the proposal would be mulled over in the foundation, but then their team would move to Geneva with some external consultants, and so could I make myself available for a day to answer any questions. Dr Don Hopkins from the Carter Centre was recruited to assist the Gates team to evaluate and critique the proposal – with invitees from the WHO.

I have not yet mentioned the WHO. Dr Lorenzo Savioli and Dr Dirk Engels had been with me all the way during the previous fact-finding year in Africa, introducing me to the various countries' WHO representatives, and helping develop the pre-proposal and contributing to the final proposal.

Unfortunately, there were others in the organization that felt that the funding should not go to the nascent SCI but would be better channelled

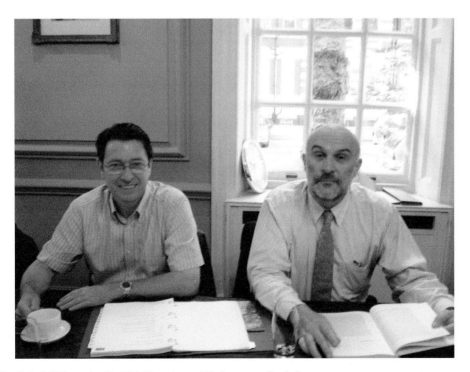

Fig. 6.3. SCI board – Dr Dirk Engels and Dr Lorenzo Savioli.

through the WHO itself. I was ready to set up shop within WHO because I was keen to work with them, but we could not agree how that could happen (my advanced age was a barrier, too – WHO retirement age was 62 and I was already perilously close to that age). Lorenzo and Dirk supported me as did David Heymann, their Director, and again, with these individuals on board the proposal went in with their blessing.

The eventual WHO support, then and ever since, has made SCI what it is today with more and more treatments delivered. Without them there would not be a success story to write about.

Where to Base the Project?

Another hurdle presented itself. If we were successful with this $34 million, where would the project be based? It became obvious that the Harvard School of Public Health was an inappropriate home for this grant. Their bureaucracy would not allow us to do what we had proposed to the foundation. Harvard, as I understood it, could not award sub-grants to anyone other than a Harvard staff member, and we and Gates Foundation wanted to have a significant research component which funded Africans to conduct research. Michael Reich and I pondered this problem and eventually took advice from a mediator. The questions we asked were: (i) Could it work at Harvard? (ii) Who should be the principal investigator? and (iii) Was there an alternative that would work better? It looked like an impossible situation, but fortunately for me, Michael (with superb timing) was offered a fantastic opportunity within Harvard which would preclude him from spending much time on schistosomiasis and even less time in Africa, so he let me 'run with the ball'. We agreed it would be better all round if I was principal investigator (PI) and I took it away from Harvard and based myself nearer to Africa.

But where should I take it? (All this was before we had actually secured the award by the way – they were worrying times.) If we could not base the programme in Africa, then I really wanted to be based in the UK – I felt that if SCI was to work, I and, eventually, several staff would need to spend a lot of time in Africa, and Boston is two overnight flights from Africa while the UK is only one. As I had already worked out, it is possible to reach every country within a day from London, either directly or via Paris. This was something which, in 2002, was not possible from anywhere in Africa, and certainly not from the USA. So I approached the London School of Hygiene and Tropical Medicine. I asked if I could apply formally to Gates for this $34 million grant and base it at LSHTM where I had been a staff member for ten years in the 1970s.

To my amazement and dismay they declined to house SCI at the LSHTM. I could not believe it; it seemed a perfect home and who would turn away $34 million? However, it transpired that Professor Brian Greenwood had a proposal in to the foundation for an equivalent sum for malaria research and control, and the LSTMH hierarchy feared (probably correctly) that the foundation might award only one, rather than both, of the large grants to one institution regardless of their quality. Remember that at that time $50,000 would have been a big grant and we were both going for over $30 million.

So Professor Greenwood did get his malaria project, which has been hugely successful, but that is another story, and I had to look elsewhere. More good luck came my way. I was fortunate at this critical time to meet Professor (now Sir) Roy Anderson, then Head of the Department of Infectious Disease Epidemiology at Imperial College London. Roy had recently moved his department from Oxford to St Mary's campus in Paddington. I had first met him some 30 years earlier at conferences and he had visited the Egypt schistosomiasis project in the 1990s when I was based in Cairo. He invited me to house SCI inside his department and smoothed the way for this to happen. How he convinced the Imperial College Research Committee to accept me to work on schistosomiasis based at St Mary's Hospital I do not know, but I suspect that his charisma, the name Bill Gates and $34 million all contributed. Thanks to Sir Roy (another to whom I am totally indebted) on 1 June 2002 I became a member of the Department of Infectious Disease Epidemiology and would remain there, expanding SCI, until retirement some 14 years later.

But I am leaping ahead – we have not been awarded the grant; we still had to pass that one-day test in Geneva.

Preparing for the Final Gates Grilling in Geneva

Michael Reich supported me magnificently because I was so tense and nervous I am sure I did not do myself justice. How do you prepare for such a grilling? Well, I decided to go to Geneva a day in advance to talk to Lorenzo and Dirk at WHO and plan how to answer the ten most difficult questions I could think of. So the morning before the Gates review I went to breakfast and was amazed to see, in the hotel restaurant, Sally Stansfield.

'What are you doing here?' she said, 'you are a day early.'

I naively explained my fiendish plan of preparation.

'What a good idea,' said Sally, 'you know what, we do not really know what to ask you, so can you give us your list of ten questions?'

What could I say? I emailed them to her and Sally ended up with the ten questions I did not want them to ask – but at least I knew what they were (she told me later that me giving her the questions removed any lingering doubts she had about the grant).

Lorenzo, Dirk, Michael and I did our preparation as best we could and the next day it all happened. The cross-examination itself was exhausting. Eight hours of critical questioning. At the end of the day, the Gates team thanked us all and invited our team out to dinner. I declined. 'I feel really low; all that is wrong with the proposal has been exposed,' I said. I really felt the day was a disaster and we had convinced no one of our capability to make a difference. Don Hopkins had been fair, but brutal, in finding all the difficulties I would face. Sally said, 'What if we told you we are ready to sign the grant award?'

So we all went out for dinner and drank some wine. We made our way back to the hotel and as we all said goodnight at the end of the evening, I remember Amy Knight, Sally's assistant, saying that the normal reaction was not usually one of joy but instead 'Holy S***t' as the realization dawned of the tasks and work ahead. However, the grant was signed and Imperial College ended up with a new staff member.

The Early Bird Catches the Worm

We really were lucky to catch Bill Gates when his foundation was relatively new.

Many people from all walks of life harbour a desire, deep down, to help their fellow human beings, especially those who are less fortunate than themselves. Some contribute their time to orphanages, some actively visit their target recipients, but many raise cash, by perhaps running a sponsored marathon, climbing a mountain or shaving their moustache. Others donate large or small sums of their own cash, but all agree that they give because they want their contribution to make a change for the better somewhere and in someone's life. Others contribute their time and expert knowledge. Scientists and researchers strive to find interventions to alleviate killer diseases: those battling to combat malaria hunt for a vaccine; likewise, billions of dollars and many man-hours are spent at the lab bench and in clinical trials testing new drugs against HIV or TB. For some conditions, and schistosomiasis is one, there are the tools, the drugs that have been discovered, but in 2000 they were not being used. I believed then that schistosomiasis could be controlled, if not eliminated, by the implementation of existing interventions and disease-control methods; more specifically, by expanding the use of the drug praziquantel, a drug discovered in the 1970s but in 2000 still not available in any country in sub-Saharan Africa. If I could buy enough praziquantel and deliver it, annually, to the millions infected with schistosomiasis in Africa, the level of suffering would surely be reduced, millions of early deaths would be avoided and productivity would be massively increased as the inhabitants of rural Africa enjoyed an improved quality of life. Just the outreach and delivery of this drug could make a massive difference.

Bill Gates realized that the simple delivery of inexpensive vaccines was extremely cost-effective and so he made his first grants in 2000 to GAVI, an organization that brought to Africa many vaccines which were used throughout the developed world. By 2020, GAVI had helped vaccinate more than 822 million children in the world's poorest countries, and by expanding their availability it prevented more than 14 million deaths due to childhood conditions such as diphtheria, measles, mumps and polio. Before the Gates Foundation, and before 2000, these vaccines and medicines were not available to, and so did not benefit, the vast majority of African rural children. For purely financial reasons, these vaccines were used only in the developed world, and the death rate in children in Africa was horrifically high.

To change this sad situation, scientists, healthcare workers, politicians, donors and educationalists all needed to develop an empathy for a deep-rooted giving and caring culture and all needed to find common ground to turn the health systems and vaccine-delivery mechanisms in Africa into efficient and far-reaching networks. A will and a mechanism were needed to reach the communities living beyond the end of the roads. GAVI was achieving this goal and I wanted to add praziquantel to the list of interventions.

During 2001 and 2002, on my fact-finding trip, I had spent many weeks in numerous countries in sub-Saharan Africa, and they were, for the most part, successful weeks, mainly, I believe (and some kind people have said as much) because I was so enthusiastic about my objectives. Another contributing factor was the respectful attitude and rapport I managed to achieve with African political leaders, who would need to approve the concept; with scientists that I had known for several years and to whom we would offer support; and finally with leaders of the communities with whom we would relate. I felt very strongly that I did not want to present SCI with a top-down, heavy-handed approach, which I perceived to be common practice by donor-government officials and some non-governmental organizations (NGOs) in the north towards African nations and nationals. I vowed to myself not to be condescending.

Having picked up some (and by that I mean a little) French, Arabic and Swahili along the way (not nearly enough), I felt ready for anything.

7 Establishing SCI – The Early Days, 2002–2003

Homeward Bound

Moving back to the UK meant a significant change in lifestyle. Moving from Khartoum to Cairo in 1988, I expected to give up playing squash and cricket and writing pantomimes, which had been my main source of non-work entertainment in Khartoum. In Cairo, although I did continue to play a lot of squash, golf became my main game, and I became very active in Rotary where I served as a founder member, and then, in 1994, as President of the Cairo Cosmopolitan Rotary Club. For many years I was the main fundraiser – Master of Ceremonies at Rotary dinners – and every week acted as Sergeant-at-Arms, making members laugh while relieving them of small amounts of money for imaginary misdemeanours. I did wonder, briefly, whether, in my new role, I would manage any time for Rotary and golf back in the UK.

In November 2001, Margie and I flew to the UK to buy a house, and after a tense week of hunting we found a perfect house within our price range in Chalfont St Giles, Buckinghamshire. The vendor was a highly skilled carpenter who had rebuilt a bungalow and converted it into a three-bedroomed chalet-type house using a lot of oak from a tree blown over during the recent UK hurricane. With the wood he built wardrobes, cupboards and the most beautiful oak kitchen. Sadly, as he neared completion, his domestic problems meant he had to sell the house to complete his divorce. We negotiated a wonderful, mutually convenient plan with the vendor. We would buy the house at the asking price, but would not take possession until five months later, in May 2002, when we finally left Egypt. In the meantime, we would allow him to live in it and his 'rent' would be to finish the upstairs rooms to our specifications, including a refit of a small bedroom as an office. The deal was done and we returned to Cairo to pack up and leave, not an easy task after 14 years.

The last few months were busy and not without problems, however – I had been diagnosed with an enlarged prostate. I was advised that I needed a transurethral resection of the prostate (TURP) and so decided to return to UK to have the operation rather than go into hospital in Cairo. I was operated on in the Royal Free Hospital in North London by the resident prostate specialist there who turned out to be an Egyptian surgeon. While I was recovering

© Fenwick, Norris and McCall 2022. *A Tale of a Man, a Worm and a Snail:*
The Schistosomiasis Control Initiative (A. Fenwick *et al.*)
DOI: 10.1079/9781786392558.0007

he came into the ward and asked me what I was doing for Christmas. He said, 'You have prostate cancer and we need to take your prostate out'. Yes, he had an excellent bedside manner! He assured me that his success rate was very high and as there are few side-effects, many of his patients were able to continue with a normal married life afterwards.

In the meantime, Margie had arranged a surprise 60th birthday party back in Cairo for me for February 2002 with my three daughters flying over to attend. The party was cancelled and instead we arranged for me to have a second opinion in Boston using my 'Harvard connection'. I spent my 60th birthday in Boston with Margie, Michael Reich and his wife Barbara, Dave Taylor – a Zimbabwean friend of Margie's now resident in the Boston area – and Nicola Sarn, whom I had known in Sudan when she was an infant and who was also, coincidentally, living there. When I visited the surgeon, who came highly recommended, he sat me down and discussed the risks and rewards of a prostate removal and reckoned that, on balance, his opinion was that I should not have my prostate removed because my cancer had a low-grade Gleason score, and in his words, 'I am almost certain something else will get you before prostate cancer does'. I have been fortunate, because I am currently 79. I am still waiting to see which gets me first.

From Boston we flew back to Cairo to pack up ready to leave in April for the UK.

Actually, to say we were both going to pack is slightly inaccurate because, much to Margie's irritation, I escaped the worst of the packing. Instead, in March, I went to Las Vegas to see my youngest daughter, Helen, get married to Darren Baker in the little church where many famous couples, including Elvis Presley, have been married.

Helen was my second daughter to be married. The eldest daughter, Janet, had married Kevin Stansfield just before she qualified as a medical doctor from St Thomas's.

I travelled with my other daughter, Gill, and her boyfriend Ben Cooke (now husband); we hired a limousine to take us to the church, a wedding dress for Helen and an Al Capone suit for Darren. Although I was only in Las Vegas for about 48 hours, I did manage a once-in-a-lifetime session in one of the hotel casinos, a massive collection of card tables, roulette wheels and slot machines. I enjoy a gamble but have no wish to return to that atmosphere.

I was back in Cairo for April, my last month, and the many farewells which are standard for expatriates leaving a country and moving on. The crates were packed and shipped and the day came for us to leave. Our move back from Cairo was made even less easy by the fact that we had two cats which we wanted to bring back to the UK (Jasper, our Siamese, and Polly, a calico cat), which meant six months in quarantine. We really wanted to avoid the mandatory six months' quarantine in the UK and came up with an alternative solution; we gave them rabies injections in Cairo and flew with them, business class, to Paris, the cats in cages at our feet and not in the hold thanks to Margie's powers of persuasion. There the cats waited out their time in a luxurious cat motel while the rabies injection was confirmed as effective and they could get cat passports. Six months after dropping the cats off in

Paris, we drove through the Euro tunnel to collect them, placing them in special transport cages to bring them back to the UK. It was scary, stressful (more red tape) but worth it.

Starting the New Job – the New Routine

On 1 June 2002 I reported for work at Imperial College. Professor Anderson introduced me to the head of the Epidemiology Division in the Faculty of Medicine, Professor Paul Elliott, and I became 'legal' at Imperial College. When the first cheque for $5 million arrived from the Bill and Melinda Gates Foundation, I became rather more popular as well.

For the first few months I left for work every morning in our beautiful new car – a bright red Jaguar – but driven to Gerrards Cross station by Margie so she was mobile during the day (public transport was not an option for getting anywhere in Chalfont St Giles). It's unthinkable now but I caught the 7.02 am train every day and returned about 7 pm to be picked up by my loving chauffeur again. Eventually, these early mornings took their toll on Margie and one evening when I returned home, I was presented with a newspaper on the table with a ring around an advertisement: 'For Sale – one small car – one elderly owner – excellent condition, low mileage'. Well, I can take a subtle hint, and two hours later I was the proud owner of a means of getting to and from the station. Margie could finally savour her morning cup of tea in bed and in the evening a glass of wine whilst waiting for me to get home.

Time for Reflection

I joined the college, immodestly and arrogantly thinking that I had enough experience and background in management, financial matters and dealing with personnel, not to mention in the field of schistosomiasis. Also, I knew how to partner with people in Africa, having spent five years working on parasitic diseases in Tanzania, 17 in Sudan, and 15 in Egypt. But I still had lots to learn. I had returned to the UK to establish the SCI and integrate it into the Department of Infectious Disease Epidemiology within the Faculty of Medicine at Imperial College of Science, Medicine and Technology in London.

I had promised to lecture, as required, on my area of expertise, aiming to inspire an up-and-coming generation of parasitologists, and tasked myself with promoting global health. A new 'sub-plot' ambition was born – to make sure that the medical students in the UK would qualify as doctors knowing about the parasitic diseases of tropical Africa. I think I was insanely driven as SCI started – and making SCI a success was my main priority. I dare not fail the foundation, the college and all those who had supported my campaign.

So the work began. I remember sending a five-page report to Sally after six months and being reprimanded. Their response was, 'All we want is a sentence to tell Bill in the elevator – and a postcard when you have finished'. That did not last long because as the Gates Foundation grew, so did the bureaucracy, but it was nice while it lasted.

Settling into Imperial College

First steps – finding the staff

I was given a free hand by my head of department Roy Anderson. I started by employing a personal assistant, Kieran Bird, who transferred from another position in the college. Fiercely loyal and ambitious (he studied at night for an MBA so he could become our office manager), he would willingly take on any task I asked of him. He also proved to be valuable because he interacted well with Peter Clark, the DFID officer who was assigned to the SCI finances after 2007, until we appointed a more senior and fully qualified accountant. That post arose when the SCI finances grew to an annual budget of approaching £20 million in 2013.

The next post I needed to fill was Deputy Director, and for this position I selected someone I knew who had so many of the skills I lacked. By chance, Howard Thompson, OBE, who I knew from Egypt, was due to retire (age 60, same age as me) from the British Council. He had served in many countries and learned the language for each, and was a proven excellent administrator. His skills were not in science or parasitology, but he complemented me brilliantly in communications, report writing and project management, and as a French speaker he was able to oversee our West Africa operations. We went together to Mali, Niger and Burkina Faso to establish the treatment programmes in each country and, in fact, started a collaborative programme with all three countries working together to combat schistosomiasis and soil-transmitted helminths (STH) by their local ministries of health and education. Howard supervised the work of the local programme managers, Dr Moussa Sacko and Dr Mamadou Traore in Mali, Dr Amadou Garba in Niger and Dr Seydou Touré in Burkina Faso.

Howard, Kieran and I set up in offices in the Bays, an old warehouse on the banks of the Regent's Canal – a dead-end branch from Little Venice to Paddington. I remember watching out of my window as moorhens hatched

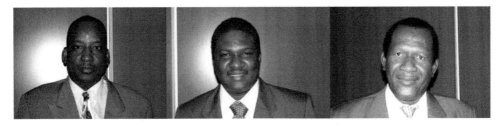

Fig. 7.1. (left to right) Seydou Touré, Amadou Garba and Moussa Sacko.

their chicks and then watching in horror as the chicks disappeared, one by one, presumably victims of a heron predator.

One really important positive step for SCI was when Roy Anderson brought Professor Joanne Webster from Oxford to the department in Imperial in 2003, and she became the SCI's Head of Research. Joanne was incredible over 12 years, never wavering in her support for SCI and standing in for me as acting director during periods of absence. Joanne was a star researcher at Imperial.

As the programme expanded, we appointed several country programme managers. The very first we hired was Dr Lynsey Blair, a new post-doc from Oxford. One of the best early memories of being Director of SCI was being able to telephone Lynsey after the interview and tell her she had been successful. She was so thrilled I think she was in tears – I know I was – and as I write this (2021), Lynsey is still with SCI and is now Director of Implementation handling a budget of over £5 million per year and overseeing treatment of over 40 million children and adults every year in 18 countries.

Our other first programme managers were Dr Albis Gabrielli, a medical doctor from Italy, who joined us to cover French–speaking countries alongside Howard, and Fiona Fleming, who during the next 18 years gained a PhD for her work and promotion to be Director of Monitoring, Evaluation and Research, a position she still holds. Albis moved on to WHO as an NTD expert based in their eastern Mediterranean region and then moved back to WHO headquarters in Geneva. He was succeeded by Elisa Bosque-Oliva. Both Albis and Elisa were amazing programme managers for West Africa and their contributions made sure that all three countries' programmes quickly expanded to national coverage.

Friendship brings another member of staff

We acquired Pedro Gazzinelli, a young Brazilian parasitologist in a roundabout way. In 2001, 30 years after leaving for Sudan and Egypt, I finally returned to Tanzania – this time with Margie – to view game in Ngorongoro Crater and Serengeti. On the way to Zanzibar from Serengeti we flew in a small plane to Arusha and stayed a couple of nights so that I could revisit my old haunts. Margie asked about Donough, my best man at my first wedding. I had lost touch with him, but of course remembered the family coffee estate he and his sisters owned.

We tried the telephone numbers we had but they did not work and so we decided to take a taxi from our hotel to the estate. The taxi driver said he knew Mringa Coffee Estate and would take us there for 28,000 Tanzania shillings, which did seem rather expensive. I dredged my memory for my Swahili and bargained him down to 14,000 shillings ('Shillingi kumi na nne elfu'). As we drove off he complemented me on my Swahili and asked where I had learned it.

'Here, in Arusha, I said.'
'When was that?' he asked.

I replied, 'Sitini na sita' ([19]66)

'What is your name?'

I replied, 'Alan.'

'Alan Fenwick?' he asked? 'Don't you remember me? I am Juma. I was your driver at TPRI in 1968.'

How weird was that? He proceeded to tell me that all my technicians were dead, but he was good...he still charged me 14,000 shillings for the trip to Mringa!

When we reached the farm, we drove up the long, straight road to the main house and Donough came to the gate to see who was driving up at 6 pm. He recognized me, hugged me like the old friends that we were and promptly invited us back for dinner the next night. He and his Brazilian wife, Beia, had plans for the evening which they couldn't alter. We accepted and made new friends immediately. Since then we have met up in the UK and kept in touch. Donough and Beia now live in Brazil where he farms.

But the point of this story is that a few years after the 2001 visit I got an e-mail from Donough to say that Beia's nephew Pedro Gazzinelli was graduating as a parasitologist in Brazil and wanted to specialize in schistosomiasis. Could Pedro and I meet up? Was there an opportunity with SCI? I arranged to see Pedro at the next annual ASTMH meeting and then he came over to the UK with Donough and Beia for a formal SCI interview. The timing was most fortunate because we desperately needed a Portuguese speaker to visit Mozambique and supervise the control programme, and then to evaluate the control measures in the Pemba region where *S. mansoni* was rampant. Pedro produced amazing results with acceptance of treatment in school-aged children and reduction in prevalence and intensity of infection.

The SCI Technical and Advisory Board appointments

The next task was to appoint a one-off Technical Committee to help select the countries for our programme. The experts we recruited included Roy Anderson, Don Bundy (from the World Bank) and Neils Christiansen (Director of the Danish Bilharzia Laboratory (DBL)). When this committee met and selected the SCI countries as described below, their work was done. To serve SCI and the Gates Foundation in the longer term, an expert Advisory Board was appointed as a condition of the Gates award. This board was to meet annually to review our working practices and evaluate our results. Because of the size of the grant, $34 million, the college senior management were keen to be involved since they knew very little about me. I was happy that they wished to be involved and offered to appoint three persons to the Advisory Board from the college – Sir Roy Anderson (who chaired it for 15 years), Tony Cannon, the then Director of Finance, and the Principal of the Faculty of Medicine, Sir Leszek Borysiewicz.

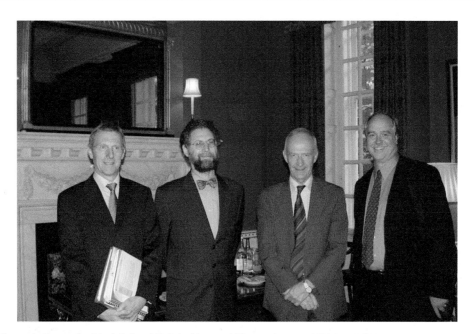

Fig. 7.2. Steve Smith, Michael Reich, Howard Thompson and Richard Olds.

We then invited two individuals from the WHO as observers – Dr David Heymann and Lorenzo Savioli (Director of the newly formed NTD department). Sally Stansfield was the representative from the Gates Foundation; and Dr Niels Christiansen was also invited onto the board because his organization was to run the small research grants section of SCI. For specific schistosomiasis expertise, Dr Ade Lucas from Nigeria and Drs Joe Cook and Richard Olds from the USA were recruited to the board. Finally, Professor Michael Reich from Harvard School of Public Health kindly maintained his interest and support to SCI by accepting to join the board.

Over an eight-year period the advisory board remained reasonably constant, with David Heymann standing down when he left WHO and Sally Stansfield handing over when she was replaced as our Gates project officer by Dr David Brandling Bennett, and later Dr Julie Jacobson. When Tony Cannon retired from the college, his successor, Andrew Murphy, and then Richard Viner, represented college finance.

Professor Steve Smith joined the board when he became Dean of the Faculty of Medicine. When the Gates funding finally ended after eight years, the whole board resigned and were replaced by a new board which, in 2010, consisted of Sir Roy Anderson and Lorenzo Savioli, who stayed on, joined by new blood Peter Dranfield, bringing his business expertise; Justine Frain, bringing expertise from big pharma (GSK); David Crompton, a retired director of the Molteno Institute in Cambridge; Lord Andrew Stone; David Heymann, who rejoined in his capacity within Public Health UK; and Stuart Smith, founder of a charity named Developing World Health.

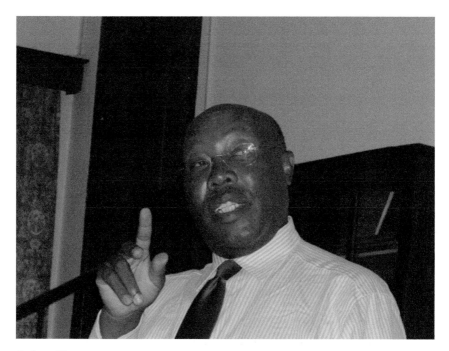

Fig. 7.3. Sam Zaramba.

We have also been honoured to have Ugandan Director General of the Ministry of Health Dr Sam Zaramba (an old friend and longtime supporter) join our board to bring an African perspective to their deliberations. David Rollinson from the Natural History Museum joined, as did Professor Joanne Webster after her transfer from Imperial College to the Royal Veterinary College.

This board was only dissolved when SCI finally left Imperial College in 2019, but that's a subject for Chapter 20.

In 2012, the Olympic Games were held in London and in celebration the then Prime Minister David Cameron in conjunction with Lord Ara Darzi hosted a dinner at the Guildhall to which ministers of health from countries attending the games were invited. The work of Imperial College and SCI was highlighted at the event and so I, too, was invited. By chance, I was sat next to Lord Andrew Stone, a peer who had been awarded the honour for his work at Marks & Spencer and for assisting Tony Blair during his period as prime minister. Lord Stone and I discussed the health programmes in Africa and we exchanged cards and he promised to meet again. He later invited me to visit the House of Lords and we have met up several times since. He was full of ideas and on the board of several charities including medical and funding organizations, and so I invited him to join the Advisory Board of SCI, where he served until 2016. Knowing him was a great experience and pleasure. His contributions to board discussions and his support for NTDs in general, and schistosomiasis in particular, in debates in the House of Lords were invaluable and greatly appreciated.

Setting up three operational units

In operational terms, the SCI established two core units in Imperial College London: an implementation unit, headed by myself, and a research unit led by Professor Joanne Webster. A third unit, the Grants Unit, was established to fund schistosomiasis research projects in Africa and this was managed by Michael Reich, Professor of Public Health Policy at the Harvard School of Public Health, and Neils Christiansen from DBL. The implementation unit was responsible for targeted financial and technical support for each national partnership programme, plus financial oversight, contract management, and procurement and distribution of praziquantel. The operational research unit was responsible for development and oversight of all the operational research programmes, monitoring and evaluation, and communication and dissemination of findings. The grants unit solicited and reviewed research grant proposals from African researchers (who all formed a collaboration with northern counterparts), and the intention was to award several $40,000 grants. Scott Gordon, who had helped prepare the original proposal, stayed on at Harvard to provide day-to-day supervision of the research award process.

The Research Challenge and DBL, Copenhagen and Building Capacity

In tune with the principle of strengthening governments and healthcare systems within Africa, the UK and the USA research scientists now aim to partner with in-country institutions and share funding for their research and development with local resources.

The reason we were keen to have DBL as part of SCI from the outset was that, back then, they already had decades of experience in capacity building, working in true partnership with several institutions in sub-Saharan Africa.

Almost all research in African institutions had been funded by grants from, and driven by agendas of, the developed world – often with resident expatriate researchers. Funded by Danish Aid (DANIDA), since 1964, DBL had tried hard to change this attitude and build a strong operational platform for African universities and institutions to run their own work. A case in point was the Ugandan Vector Control Division (VCD) in Kampala which operated as an arm of the Ministry of Health – important work – but they were not gaining recognition internally because of their reliance on foreign funding and scientists. DBL support changed this and enabled VCD to develop its own strong visibility and identity within Uganda.

Neils and DBL were thus well-placed to help SCI organize and run the research arm of the Gates grant known as the Schistosomiasis Research Programme (SRP). This ran from 2005 to 2007, awarding relatively small (up to $40,000) grants to African principal investigators. These grants were focused on strengthening operational research so that we could optimize the effectiveness of services.

It is noteworthy that both the Wellcome Trust and the Liverpool School of Tropical Medicine have also followed this model, promoting local capacity development and training of African scientists. An even newer programme awarding grants to Africans run by a consortium of European foundations (headed by the Volkswagen Foundation) has led to more local research into NTDs. SCI has always stressed that the control programmes it supports are owned and run by local teams.

SCI's Implementation Principles

In each of the six partner countries, the ministry of health was asked to appoint a local national co-ordinator who would be the key link between the ministries and the SCI. Our support would operate through small teams of trained health workers from each district responsible to the national co-ordinator.

We recognized that in a programme involving school-based treatments, teachers need to be fully informed about the programmes and convinced that providing their schoolchildren with this medication is worthwhile. The teachers have an incredible influence in the community and, of course, over the children and so SCI factored in regular training and refresher workshops for them. To do this, SCI would train central ministry of health staff who then travelled to the districts to train the district health staff who, in turn, then trained teachers in the targeted schools. These days you would call them 'train-the-trainer workshops'.

Most importantly, I believed that we had to develop SCI to be perceived by everyone involved, especially local populations, as a long-term investment over many years rather than a flighty attempt to solve a problem temporarily and depart. For this reason, the proposal to the Gates Foundation had articulated that the objectives of the SCI were to establish long-term, sustainable intervention programmes with a strong well-trained local infrastructure. These key strategies, which have guided the project, are what has made the SCI so successful.

When we therefore approached the countries, we offered to the ministers that our aims were to assist the local ministries to strengthen existing national control programmes by providing the necessary medicines (praziquantel and albendazole), supported by financial and technical assistance to map the distribution and deliver the treatments.

Where did albendazole come from? Well, simply, our technical committee reminded us that almost everyone infected with schistosomiasis was also infected with STH, which all could be flushed out with a single pill of albendazole, and their recommendation (which we quickly accepted) was that while reaching out to dose people with praziquantel we should add in one tablet of albendazole – a tablet which should cost us just 2 pence.

Our aim would be to create an improved awareness of schistosomiasis and STH and their consequences amongst local communities and national health professionals, decision makers and international organizations. The implementation we would support would ensure control programmes were effective and sustainable, alleviating immediate suffering and improving the quality of life of the rural populations. I was confident that by providing annual treatments people would feel the benefit, and the word would spread, thus creating a demand for ongoing treatment which would be essential to stop the disease from escalating again.

Above all, the SCI would go to great lengths to ensure that local agencies involved in schistosomiasis control did not see us as an uninvited and interfering guest: SCI would strive to work with agencies already in existence and be seen at the local level. Long term, we aimed to bring in the resources so that we could expand in any country which requested our presence, and to advocate for the initiation and expansion of national control efforts to create a more supportive environment for control programmes at the national level.

However, there was one requirement to keep in mind: the Gates Foundation stressed that SCI make a valuable contribution to research and capacity building. Despite substantial findings through the SRP in Egypt, as health-management programmes expand in size, new and more beneficial solutions and methods emerge. The basic science which needed to be included in our work related to looking out for any development of resistance on a phenotypic and genotypic level by close monitoring and evaluation. It became a mainstay of the SCI to conduct research and evaluate the tools, techniques and approaches that would make it easier to manage sustainable control programmes. We would then publish our findings to disseminate the information gathered and any lessons learned. This was a condition of the grant, but also a condition of Imperial College when accepting SCI because of their reputation as a college of research excellence. Professor Joanne Webster joined SCI with the express ambition to fulfil those expectations.

Praziquantel Becomes Available at a Lower Price

My determination to launch an African continent-wide campaign could not have been timed better. The turn of the century also coincided with significant changes in the praziquantel market in terms of manufacturing capacity and a significant reduction in price. It is a great injustice that even when effective drugs exist to treat serious infectious diseases, it is unlikely that the neediest patients in the poorest countries will have access to the medication, or that they will have access to a well-equipped and staffed healthcare centre to deliver the medication. Several reasons existed at the time, including lack of money, poor infrastructure, political unrest, lack of epidemiological data, lack of realization of the need, poor logistics, or any combination of these or other factors. Enough praziquantel was needed for an annual regimen on a national scale. However, when, by 2000, the price had dropped by over 90% to less than ten cents per tablet, the treatment of schistosomiasis became an attractive and cost-effective proposition. With SCI having funds to purchase praziquantel, more pharmaceutical companies and formulators started to produce the tablets and the market competition drove the price downwards.

(The selling price stood at 8 cents per tablet in 2005, but then started to rise with inflation.) If SCI was to treat as many children as we wanted to, praziquantel and albendazole had to be purchased and distributed, and due to the large scale of the operation, I hoped that SCI would be in a prime position to negotiate prices based on economies of scale.

Technical Committee Selects the First Countries to Support

Making hard choices

When it was signed, the final value of the funds awarded to the SCI was US$28.6 million to provide technical and financial support for the development of national control programmes in sub-Saharan countries. A smaller parallel grant of US$5 million was awarded to WHO to establish the Partners for Parasite Control (PPC), with which SCI would interact. Together we had funds to provide the 'proof of principle' that would encourage other countries in sub-Saharan Africa to plan campaigns against schistosomiasis and STH and persuade other donors that such campaigns were feasible and economically cost-effective. We needed to determine how many countries we could work in with the amount of funding at our disposal, and we needed to choose which countries they would be. We needed to budget for each selected country for five years, and to decide how much of the funding would be spent on purchasing the drugs we needed and how much to retain for funding the implementation, monitoring and evaluation. Finally, we had to decide on staffing needs to achieve our targets. I realized that I would win a lot of friends in the successful countries, but sadly, I stood to lose friends in those countries which I had visited and had encouraged to develop proposals, but which were not selected.

So now, when established and ready to start treatments, SCI was faced with the unenviable and daunting task of having to select a handful of countries in which to implement control of schistosomiasis and STH.

Sub-Saharan Africa covers a geographical area of 24.3 million km^2 and according to 2006 World Bank figures was home to 770.3 million people. WHO published data suggested that over 25% of this population were infected with schistosomiasis, with an equal number living at risk. The 42 countries and six island nations that comprise the region together represent the poorest area in the world due to a mixture of harsh physical and climatic conditions, limited resources, some economic mismanagement, political instability, corruption and inter-tribal conflict.

Consultation with our technical committee and our partners, the WHO, confirmed that we should develop and implement a strict selection process, initially choosing those countries that appeared to have a high prevalence of infection *and*, because of good governance, were the most likely to speedily facilitate the implementation of a schistosomiasis/STH control programme. My initial suggestion was to select four countries, because if the programme worked we would easily be able to convince a wide range of donors that it was worth investing millions of dollars or pounds in the project and we would be able to expand across the region.

The advances which would help us meet these ambitions were, in addition to the cheaper medicine, some new low-cost technologies aimed at facilitating large-scale treatment programmes. These technologies had already been trialled and field tested in Africa (Utzinger *et al.*, 2015). First, self-reported questionnaires asking about blood in urine for schoolchildren were proved to be reasonably accurate in assessing prevalence of infection for *S. haematobium* (Coulibaly *et al.*, 2013). Then, a height/dose pole had been developed to determine the dose of praziquantel needed based on height as a proxy for weight of children (Montressor *et al.*, 2001). Finally, a GIS with remote sensing and satellite imaging had been designed to predict from satellite images the ecological zones where schistosomiasis was likely to be found.

There was no other way to ensure that the most appropriate countries and governments were selected than to take the time to personally visit the countries again. I revisited the ten countries in sub-Saharan Africa that were quoted in our proposal and invited each of them to prepare more detailed proposals for SCI. However, I had to warn them that our funding would probably only be enough to fund four country programmes. The criteria that would be used for selection would include: that WHO judged them to have viable national plans for schistosomiasis control, preferably demonstrated by the countries already having conducted planning workshops for schistosomiasis control. The Gates Foundation understandably required an assurance that any country which received support were willing to place enough priority to schistosomiasis relative to other diseases, and that resources received would be made available at the right time and to the right people through the ministries of health and education.

We issued invitations to submit proposals to five countries in East Africa (Kenya, Malawi, Tanzania, Uganda and Zambia) and five in West Africa (Burkina Faso, Cameroon, Mali, Niger and Nigeria), and the WHO played a major role in helping with the preparation phase. I held meetings with the directors of health services and their associates in each country and, frankly, it came as no surprise that none of these countries had really prioritized schistosomiasis as a serious public health issue that needed more attention, and had not allocated resources to roll out mass treatment programmes. Each country had some ministry of health staff who knew these treatments were needed, but they each were woefully short of funding for all their health work, and so, in setting priorities, schistosomiasis and STH did not reach very high on the list. The bare facts were that schistosomiasis, de-worming, school health and the other parasitic diseases were not even mentioned in any of these countries' five-year national health plans.

Despite this low priority, the ten countries listed above did agree that they would like to host an externally funded control programme and were willing to prepare and submit a proposal. I was convinced that the ten offered the best chance of conducting an effective programme, and that all of them would collaborate and use our SCI resources to demonstrate the principle that mass treatment programmes (aka MDA) can be efficiently managed and would reduce prevalence and then morbidity from infection. Essentially, they were countries that showed a welcoming interest in what SCI had to offer, and had apparently effective, trustworthy leadership high up in their government.

Selecting the countries – can we support six instead of four?

In East Africa, Uganda, Tanzania and Zambia were chosen. The East African countries have many features in common but are spread over a wide geographical area stretching far to the north and the south of the region and, as such, needed to be treated separately. But that left just one more country.

When it came to the crunch, so difficult was it to turn away countries that the technical committee recommended to the advisory board that six countries were supported. The way we managed to add the two extra countries was to consider three countries as one entity. They were in West Africa: Mali, Burkina Faso and Niger, and they were selected because they all shared similar ecological settings, they were manageably small, and agreed to work as a regional entity where appropriate. These factors were important to SCI and WHO, and so despite their different political systems, they were considered as the 'fourth country'.

The saddest loss for me was when we decided that we had to limit our activities to six countries; we did not select Cameroon as one of the six. I have never really been forgiven by the wonderful Dr Louis Albert Tchuem-Tchuente who had worked very hard to prepare a strong proposal, and he was supported by his minister of health.

I am sure he blames me, but actually Cameroon was not chosen *despite* my efforts on their behalf to the technical committee, not *because* of me. One of the committee felt strongly that Cameroon was too difficult a country to work in at that time.

As a postscript, the countries we did not include in our programme have all now been supported. In 2006, Cameroon was included in the RTI bid to USAID and has been treated annually ever since. Kenya was adopted by the UK-based Children's Investment Fund Foundation and their programmes were soon up and running implemented by the Partnership for Child Development, also based at Imperial College. Malawi was added to SCI's portfolio as soon as DFID funding came on stream in 2010. Nigeria, of course, is huge and several different states in Nigeria have received targeted support from different donor agencies. The Carter Center supported initially Plateau and Nasara states, but expanded to include eight others. The 2012 DFID funding included support for three more states in Nigeria implemented by Sightsavers and SCI in collaboration.

The six selected countries were invited to meet at a workshop held at Imperial College in July 2003 in London. The Minister of Health and the Director General of Health for Uganda jointly chaired the meeting. They

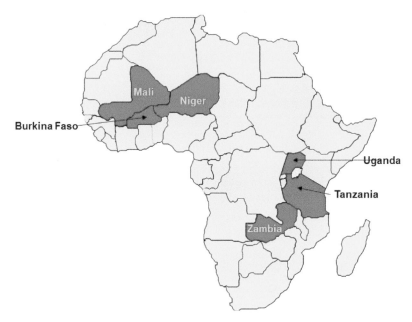

Fig. 7.4. SCI-selected countries, west and east. (After SCI, adapted by Wendie Norris)

reviewed the Ugandan proposed national plans to assist the other countries to develop their plans in detail. The countries which submitted their proposals but were not selected because of the limited resources were Cameroon, Kenya, Malawi and Nigeria.

Uganda seemed to be ready to go

I was personally most encouraged by Uganda, which had already taken substantial strides towards planning their own schistosomiasis control programme, even though they did not have the funding to implement the programme. It also appeared to be the strongest country in terms of political support and the existing infrastructure of the health management system. The programme manager there was a most engaging character, Dr Narcis Kabatereine, and several more junior district health officers had already started training with WHO, providing the perfect springboard from which to launch the SCI.

Creating an Active Praziquantel Market in Africa

Another of our early tasks, after country selection, was to decide how to procure and deliver praziquantel. Thanks to the grant from the Gates Foundation, the SCI held a very strong position enabling it to purchase praziquantel on an unprecedented scale, thereby utilizing the dual pricing advantages of competition and economy of scale. Through careful use of its procurement opportunities, the SCI strategically shaped the market for praziquantel in Africa and stimulated competition among different companies. Effectively, the SCI did what every marketer dreams of doing: it created an active marketplace for a product where none existed before. And even though the SCI was initially buying less than 20 million tablets a year, a competitive market was formed (more about this in Chapter 12).

After a tender process in 2003/4, SCI was able to procure praziquantel through Shin Poong, a for-profit private pharmaceutical company in South Korea; the International Dispensary Association (IDA), a not-for-profit pharmaceutical procurement agency based in Holland; and Pharmchem, a UK-based supplier who used a pharmaceutical formulator in India called Flamingo. A later tender enabled two African companies, TPI and Shelys, to also formulate the drug for SCI.

SCI purchased much of its praziquantel from Shin Poong and the IDA for the duration of the Gates Foundation grant (2003–2007), and albendazole from GSK's approved suppliers in India.

In addition, we had the good fortune to receive donated supplies from a third source, MedPharm, a US pharmaceutical company. MedPharm's donation comes with a unique story. In 2004, SCI and WHO were approached by Andrew Koval, CEO of MedPharm to consider whether SCI's objectives and activities were suitable for the company's drug donation programme to the developing world. In the donation programme offered to SCI, MedPharm would buy drugs from European and Indian formulators using funds from a Canadian NGO (Escarpment Biosphere Foundation [EBF]) through the Canadian Humanitarian Trust. These funds came from the public who then received tax credits to the value of the drugs purchased. This mechanism benefitted from an apparent loophole in the tax regulations which allowed the praziquantel value claimed to be at Ontario prices rather than actual prices. EBF was therefore offering tax relief at $1 per tablet and yet purchasing from Indian suppliers at 8 cents a tablet.

In February 2004, MedPharm donated 680,000 praziquantel and one million albendazole tablets to the SCI for use in Zanzibar and Zambia. In June 2004, MedPharm pledged to donate a further 13.7 million praziquantel tablets, which were delivered by the end of 2004, then added a further 12 million tablets in 2005. MedPharm suggested it could repeat the donation annually for the life of the original SCI project (through to 2007). Sadly, for SCI and the children of Africa, the Canadian tax authorities changed their rules, closing the tax loophole, and the benefit of these donations disappeared.

Getting Started in Uganda

Uganda was nominated as the SCI flagship country and after a review of their proposal developed with and submitted by Dr Narcis Kabatereine, on behalf of Uganda, the technical committee drew up a specification of the type of parasitological data needed and the required size of statistically significant samples to be collected by each county within that country. The chosen criteria relating to data collection and sample sizes had to allow for the potential of inconsistency over a five-year period and allow for a predicted number of potential drop-outs. There was also concern over whether the given timeframe would be long enough to demonstrate sufficient reduction in infection rates as well as whether morbidity would show any improvement over this relatively short period. Despite these constraints, the basis of the monitoring and evaluation component of each treatment programme was developed (see Chapter 14). Data collection could then begin in the field in Uganda in three highly endemic districts in October 2002, and a further three districts would be started in the following spring – as soon as a memorandum of understanding could be signed.

The Memorandum Chain – Six Degrees of Separation

It is a well-established fact that we are only ever six degrees of separation away from anyone else on the planet. So it was demonstrated with the story of my first SCI country visit and the first memorandum of understanding (MoU) signing in Uganda. I arrived in Uganda in search of a signature from the minister of health on an MoU between Uganda and the SCI, Imperial College. This MoU would open the door to SCI transferring funding for a bilharzia and STH control programme in that country and lead to national coverage of treatment of over 3 million individuals with praziquantel and albendazole against schistosomiasis and STH, respectively. The in-country ministry of health national co-ordinator for bilharzia (as schistosomiasis is known in Uganda) was, as I said, Dr Narcis Kabatereine. He was an individual well known in the schistosomiasis community because from conference to conference over the years he had published results demonstrating the devastating effects of schistosomiasis in West Nile, along the shores of Lakes Victoria and Albert. His data showed incredibly high prevalence of infection and a high death rate due to *Schistosoma mansoni*. He was desperate to get treatment to millions of infected and at-risk individuals, but bilharzia was a neglected tropical disease in Uganda and no funding was available, no praziquantel was available and no treatments were administered. On learning of the success of my Gates application, he had attempted to contact the Permanent Secretary for Health on my behalf to make an appointment, but to no avail. It seemed that Dr Narcis was more famous outside Uganda than inside his own ministry of health. So I decided I would go to Uganda and stay as long as it took to track down the Permanent Secretary and/or minister himself. Treating people in Uganda was my first mission, and we wanted to start with baseline data collection as soon as possible.

In a sequence of events reminiscent of the Pied Piper of Hamelin, I collected a chain of officials *en route* to reaching the Ugandan minister of health,

MDGs and SDGs

The eight Millennium Development Goals (MDGs) of 2000 aimed to improve primary education, halve extreme poverty, improve maternal health and reduce childhood mortality as well as halt the spread of HIV/AIDS, malaria and 'other diseases' (a vague reference wherein languished NTDs) by 2015.

My colleagues and I consistently argued that these goals would never be achieved if attention was not given to the control of NTDs, as is apparent to those familiar with these infections and their consequences. Children infected with NTDs cannot work effectively in school, while women with anaemia caused by NTDs are likely to have a poor birth outcome. Fortunately, and rightly, the Sustainable Development Goals (SDGs) which superseded the MDGs now include several important goals which point directly to the NTDs.

First Steps

We determined to raise the profile of NTDs and make our case for an integrated approach to the control of the seven diseases (Lammie *et al.*, 2006). We gathered evidence for the collective global burden demonstrating that when NTDs are taken as a whole, the burden is at least the same as either malaria or TB (Hotez *et al.*, 2006, 2007). And yet, while the US government in particular, and others, had poured billions of dollars into fighting the big three, the NTDs had received a miniscule amount of funding for implementation of control and research.

Without detracting from the importance of the big three, which used to kill millions each year, we believed that using tried-and-tested strategies – existing medicines, vector control tools – and the setting of realistic goals for control, the ultimate elimination of the seven NTDs could be possibly achieved by 2030.

The Need for Integration, Collaboration and Coherence across Programmes

Support for our cause developed over time and came from a variety of sources. With SCI as the latest initiative, NGOs had pursued their own agendas and implemented treatment programmes against their 'favourite' disease (SCI being no exception concentrating on schistosomiasis). However, by 2004, the Gates Foundation, the major funder at the time, realized that these annual programmes were often targeting the same geographic areas endemic for NTDs and the same populations (preschool children or school-age children). Thus, as the programmes expanded their coverage, they increasingly tended to overlap with one another and treat the same poly-parasitized, poverty-stricken individuals.

It was realized that this situation could lead to a duplication of drug administration, even dangerous overdose of drugs, but also a significant waste of resources. Costs could be saved if drug administrations could be integrated or at least collaborate.

Equally, if the donating and implementing agencies could collaborate, the jobs for the local officials responsible for arranging MDAs would be made much easier. One NTD team in the ministries of health would improve the use of limited resources and avoid, in extreme cases, an individual being treated by four organizations with four individual medications to treat seven diseases (more about this from Chapter 15 onwards).

To encourage integration and collaboration between the implementing NGOs and ministries of health, the Gates Foundation convened a meeting to coincide with the ASTMH annual meeting. At the first two meetings, about 30 participants attended the movement towards integration. But by 2012, funded by the Gates Foundation and USAID, and hosted by Pat Lammie and his team from the Task Force for Global Health, Atlanta, the meeting had grown to accommodate 500 participants. Donors, academics, NGOs and ministry of health representatives now attend an expanded two-day meeting.

There were a number of other defining moments during this period of advocacy which contributed to the success story.

UK Commission for Africa Report 2005 Mentions NTDs

The emphasis placed on building in-country capacity has been widely echoed in international development circles, which encourage the allocation of funds and promote schemes behind existing health and education systems.

During the Blair-led Labour government in the UK (1997–2005), the UK Commission for Africa published a report in 2005 with a major call to action. The report was written by an international task force which highlighted the need for the development community to act on integrating health initiatives into local government systems. I have no idea if Tony Blair had any idea about NTDs but I do know that Miles Wickstead and Rebecca Affolder, who both contributed a great part of the report, were great supporters of SCI and the other NGOs implementing NTD control programmes. They appreciated the efforts we were making to expand the visibility of the NTDs, and supported our cause by including some excellent sentences in the report:

> …and they [the donated medicines to treat NTDs] must be delivered. But not through new initiatives. Rather, through financing that supports coherent country-led strategies for strengthening health and education systems. Donor funding has been short term, volatile and largely tied to using people and products from donor countries. Single-issue initiatives have led to the setting up of parallel systems in competition with each other, further undermining government capacity.

freshwater lake or river, the child will be exposed to the very parasite they seek to avoid.

Vector Control

As I have written in the sections on my life in Tanzania and Sudan, control of snails using chemical molluscicides, plant molluscicides or environmental measures have all been tried under various epidemiological conditions, but apparent success in killing snails has not been shown to reduce transmission, and control has proved to be short-term and expensive. However, in the context of the current global elimination strategy for schistosomiasis, it does have a role. WHO is now reinforcing snail control, focusing on discovery of new molluscicides, which are both cost-effective and low-risk to humans and the environment, and rebuilding capacity (through provision of a 2017 field manual on use of molluscicides).

Vaccines: Could there Be One for Schistosomiasis?

Development of a vaccine has regularly been proposed since the 1970s and pursued as the most likely eventual, most workable solution to widespread schistosomiasis infection. If a vaccine were available, individuals would no longer have to attend a clinic annually for praziquantel, because even if a vaccine was needed every few years, we would have removed the onus on the patient of having to comply with annual drug regimens. Unfortunately, despite many millions of dollars having been invested over many years of research into a vaccine for schistosomiasis, results have yielded nothing workable to date in terms of both long-term protection and a candidate vaccine that can be produced in large-enough quantities.

What Are We Delivering?

Praziquantel

In the case of schistosomiasis and indeed several other NTDs, the development of a vaccine has, so far, been considered an insurmountable obstacle and unlikely to be cost-effective compared to the relatively straightforward treatment schedules.

Considering the (2002) low price of praziquantel (8 cents per tablet), programmes such as those supported by SCI have met with considerable success, and with the now massive quantity of donated praziquantel, even elimination can be considered as possible without the use of a vaccine. Perhaps the delivery of praziquantel using MDA could be considered as a vaccine.

Barriers to Success

In the absence of a hygienic environment and improved education, using pharmaceutical interventions like praziquantel to control levels of infection is the most practical and immediate solution. But whereas pharmaceutical interventions on a wide scale offer an easy-to-deliver, effective solution in developed countries, they are often fraught with constraints in many parts of sub-Saharan Africa.

The constraints could be caused by the variation of infection rates. Infection rates are not homogeneous across countries or even at the village level. Variation of infection rate between villages leads to different demands for the drug. Thus, if the same amount of praziquantel is delivered to each village based on population alone there may be too much drug in one village and not enough in another. Carefully planned mapping is required to determine the detailed needs in each village or district.

More obvious difficulties in rural Africa are poor roads, blockage of roads during the rains and a lack of suitable storage. Even if the tablets are available in the local health units, persuading the villagers to comply may present formidable challenges if there is no health education and adequate preparation before the treatment days. Remote villagers may well be suspicious of a free pill distribution, and quietly hide from drug distributors. Finally, political instability or military or civil unrest will all contribute to poor compliance in a campaign.

Despite all these potential constraints, SCI believes that MDA is the best option available. We take these factors into consideration and plan for them whenever possible.

Supply chain, logistics and sustainability

The principle of carefully matching the target population and the proposed frequency of MDA to each population's need, was necessary to optimize the use of our limited resources. In the years 2003–2010, the availability of praziquantel was limited because we were buying the drug by tender. Our success in these years of the programme and our advocacy meant demand increased as more countries wanted national control programmes. Very few countries in sub-Saharan Africa had purchased praziquantel, even at the lower cost of 8–10 cents/600 mg tablet, and so at first, SCI, and then USAID, were the only sources of the medication. Before there would be any chance of a country purchasing praziquantel, the ministries of health and finance would need to be convinced of the cost-effectiveness of its use, hence the importance of the monitoring and evaluation (M&E) component of the SCI-supported programmes.

Consequently, in each of the first six countries assisted by SCI, an M&E study was carried out over the first five years to measure the success of the MDA campaign (see Chapter 14).

Public–Private Partnerships in Developing Countries

The development of praziquantel from a successful laboratory compound into a drug for human use in MDA was the first large-scale collaborative project to demonstrate the benefit of public–private partnership in drug development for poor countries. WHO's assistance and the role of Assistant Director General Dr Andrew (Rikk) Davis in helping to organize the clinical trials of praziquantel (including those I carried out in Angado village, Sudan) was critical during this phase of its development. By the mid-1990s, Bayer and E. Merck had registered the patent for praziquantel in 38 countries.

However, there was a very large stumbling-block ahead. The public–private partnership failed to effectively address the issue of access to praziquantel in poor countries. These countries could not allocate funding from their meagre health budget to purchase sufficient praziquantel to treat their at-risk population annually.

Having achieved country registration, the partnership had not taken the vital step of providing any agreement on pricing nor on distribution methods after development. The German government initially supported some use of praziquantel, by buying to fulfil the needs for large-scale field trials, but no donor government nor any government in sub-Saharan Africa could commit to buy the drug for long-term annual distribution to the millions of people who needed it. And so, from 1980 to 2002, there was never an active market – and the reason was the price and the cost of buying the quantities needed.

This experience provided important lessons about public–private partnerships: long-term access issues need to be addressed as an integral part of product development and agreements on access and price need to be explicit, written and transparent at an early stage. Because Bayer marketed praziquantel without assessing the potential market and the need for a competitive price structure, their price at $1 per tablet, $4 for an adult dose, was too high and there were no takers. Few of the 200 million people infected in sub-Saharan Africa actually possessed $4 let alone had enough to spare to buy a drug that would offer only temporary relief and require annual treatment.

Shin Poong to the Rescue

SCI was in the fortunate position that Shin Poong in Korea had made a breakthrough in praziquantel (PZQ) synthesis, which by 2004 had reduced the price per tablet to less than 8 cents and enabled our plan. We could now treat a child annually for 50 cents. For us, it meant wide-scale treatment programmes were now possible as the drug was affordable – not to the end-user but to donor and aid organizations to fund its purchase and distribution.

Shin Poong had entered the PZQ market in the 1980s. They effectively provided the breakthrough to trigger wide-scale treatment programmes (aka MDA). This encouraged local pharmaceutical companies to formulate tablets using the cheaper ingredient. For example, the Egyptian Ministry of Health purchased its praziquantel for annual MDA in 1994 from an Egyptian

pharmaceutical company, EIPICO, who used the cheaper Shin Poong ingredient (see Chapter 5). SCI not only took advantage of the reduced price but also
took note of this aspect of the supply chain and built into our plan the encour-
agement and facilitation of local supply by African companies (see Chapter 7).

Once Shin Poong agreed to provide SCI with the drug at a price per tablet of
less than 8 cents, I realized this heralded the beginning of a new era in mass treatment. The price reduction presented an opportunity that could not be missed.
Thus, in 2000, with a record of success in wide-scale treatment programmes
in Egypt behind me and 40 years research experience, I began developing my
strategy to build and expand the market (see six-point plan in Chapter 12) and
facilitate access to the drug in sub-Saharan Africa. I approached Dr Dirk Engels
and Dr Lorenzo Savioli at WHO, and they helped us implement the plan when
SCI was launched. By 2004/05, SCI was buying all the tablets that Shin Poong
could produce and the company became the leading supplier of praziquantel in
tablet form to Burkina Faso, Mali, Niger, Uganda, Tanzania and Zambia, with
tablets purchased by SCI through their Gates funding.

Will Drug Resistance to Praziquantel Develop?

Throughout my career as a deliverer of praziquantel in large quantities, I
have given this potential disaster some considerable thought and I am now
one of those who believe that resistance will take a long time to develop
(if it even can) in the case of schistosomiasis. I go into more detail, based
on research evidence, in Chapter 17 but in summary there are three main
reasons.

The first reason is the length of time it takes to complete the life cycle
and the isolation of the breeding female worm within the human host. The
opportunity for sexual reproduction with a resistant partner is limited to one.
The second reason is 'refugia', a veterinary concept that means that if not
every human is treated there will always be a mixture of susceptible worms
in the environment. Finally, and perhaps most important, is the fact that
although praziquantel-resistant worms have been developed in laboratories,
they have proved to be weak in reproducing, and in the real world these
worms have never spread.

There have been scary reports of drug failures; however, looking at the
poor cure rates reported from Senegal, which was the most vocal, I believe
the reported 'failure' of praziquantel was, in fact, due to the extreme and
unique transmission conditions there. The change in habitat brought about
by the construction of the Diama dam in the early 1980s decimated the crayfish, which used to eat the snails and this facilitated snail breeding. This led
to intense transmission and speedy re-infection for the human population,
which meant that praziquantel could not kill the worms quickly enough to
be effective. It was a scare about the drug's efficacy that proved to be false,
but the episode was a lesson that we needed to keep in mind the possibility
of resistance.

10 Across Borders – Implementing Schistosomiasis Control from East to West Africa

Few could refute that a nation's health is inextricably linked to the economic status of its population. So it comes as no surprise to find that people living on less than two dollars a day are rife with disease and can expect their lives to be short. The six countries selected for SCI support in 2003 embodied the poorest of the poor.

Poverty and Poor Health Go Together

Poverty and poor health could be attributed to any number of factors, but the overwhelming indirect factors are the hot tropical climate, a stark lack of basic education, a lack of clean water and inadequate sanitation. A lack of government funding for public services means there is very little provision of clean water, healthcare or transport in rural areas. The lack of piped-water

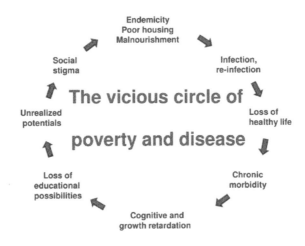

Fig. 10.1. Circle of poverty and disease (Bergquist and Whittaker, 2012).

supplies forces everyone to use open water bodies for all domestic purposes; to wash clothes and to clean cooking utensils as well as their bodies.

The lack of education reduces employment prospects and leaves the villagers unable to pay for these services themselves.

In the search for workable land and the need to supply food for their families and animals, villages tend to be sited by the edge of water bodies which are then used by the whole population for every activity – drinking, irrigation, fishing, bathing and as toilets. This same water is the source of parasite vectors which naturally leads to transmission of schistosomiasis and STH, and the breeding of the insect vectors such as mosquitoes, sandflies and blackflies.

As stated earlier, it is because of this increased and varied activity around the water source that school-age children are often the most heavily infected.

East versus West Africa – Major Differences in Characteristics

The SCI-selected countries, three in the east and three in the west of Africa, are contrasted in terms of their climatic and political influences, their demography and their language, but not in their levels of poverty. Mali, Niger and Burkina Faso in the west are ex-French colonial territories, while Tanzania, Uganda and Zambia in the east were all British before they became independent in the 1960s.

Although the six countries all share a tropical climate, each has a mixture of zones from arid to tropical forests. In the west, the three countries are aligned along an east–west axis and so occupy similar ecological zones, whereas those countries in the east lie along a north–south axis covering a wide range of latitudes above and below the equator.

Within Mali, Niger and Burkina Faso, there are three distinct climatic zones, including the Saharan zone to the north (a very arid zone with a rainfall of less than 300 mm p.a.), a Sahelian region below the desert (rainfall between 300–700 mm) and a Sudanian climatic zone in the south, which enjoys a much heavier rainfall (above 700 mm p.a.). There are no major inland lakes in the three countries but the Niger river flows through all of them, with significant tributaries. In this western region, aid programmes sometimes follow the geography of a river and its basin, so, for example, the World Bank's Senegal River Basin Aid Project addresses issues on a regional basis, using the river basin as the framework for projects involving water distribution.

In contrast, all of the eastern countries have relatively high but seasonal rainfall in most parts of the country. Indeed, during the aerial approach to Uganda's capital airport, you would be forgiven for thinking that it was an archipelago with lush green vegetation emerging from the 36,330 km^2 of extensive lake waters.

These countries all have very large lakes, with Lake Victoria (Tanzania and Uganda) and Lakes George and Albert (Uganda) being the most significant, while Zambia has Lake Kariba along its southern border. Additionally,

Uganda has the River Nile running from south to north, while Zambia has the Kariba river.

Despite the differences between the east and west regions, the six countries chosen are also characterized by the fact that developmental progress is restricted by a shortage of public funds and a wide distribution of the seven NTDs.

The Changing Face of Communication Networks in Africa

A sense of community and mutual goodwill were distinctive features of sub-Saharan societies in the 1960s, where communications and infrastructure were severely limited. In this environment, in 1966, a 150 km road trip for us could take six hours to traverse the murram roads, often with two wheels of our 4x4 navigating a ditch. And after rain, the road could well be completely impassable. It was not unusual for local people to have to walk 15 miles to a clinic, three miles for water and a mile or more to the fields where they worked or their livestock grazed. In many villages there might be one small shop, and the batteries they sell keep people in touch with regional news through local FM radio. No electricity means no light after sunset and certainly no national radio or television.

In the communication revolution since 2000, mobile phones have become commonplace due to the minimal infrastructure required to operate networks and the clever marketing by MTN and other operators. The result is that, whereas initially reaching out to people was incredibly difficult and communications often began and ended at the village boundaries, networks have sprung up, and making personal contacts with the right people has become possible and of the utmost importance.

SCI was able to use this improved technology to publicize the MDA programmes they were supporting.

Health Services in East and West Africa

Accessing local healthcare

Travel between towns and villages in Africa, even in 2002, could be tortuous and slow. Even if a road existed, few people had vehicles to use it, and if they did, fuel was limited and few could pay the price. The upshot was that even when adequate healthcare was available at central health centres, many people could not afford the time and expense to travel the distance to reach them. This is one of sub-Saharan Africa's most challenging obstacles to achieving an efficient healthcare system – that each centre, in theory, is intended to serve the population of several villages, but in practice it serves only the population who live quite close to the building.

The challenge of population dispersal

The pattern of population distribution varies between countries in the east and west and is largely driven by the availability of fresh water and fertile land to support crops and livestock. In both regions, more people live in rural locations than in cities but due to the overall poor quality of cultivable land in the western African countries, the population tends to be more widely dispersed than in the east.

When the pasture is poor, families need a larger expanse of land to support their goats, sheep and cattle, which provide the basis of their economy. The net result of this settlement pattern is that households are often located several kilometres apart and are not always concentrated into villages or small towns. Inevitably, this leads to difficulties for the provision of healthcare and education due to the problem of finding an optimum location for either a health centre or school within reasonable walking distance for the majority of people.

In terms of rainfall distribution, Uganda, Zambia and Tanzania are more fortunate than countries further west due to relatively predictable rainy seasons. This climatic pattern, and the availability of better pasture on their land to support animals, leads to a more concentrated distribution of population.

Thus, in East Africa health centres are within reach for a higher proportion of the population. Even so, the distances can still be challenging, and far enough to make access to health services difficult. Roads are being improved, and local bus services now serve more of the remote villages; but, even so, the extra transport is by no means universal or convenient for all people.

Decentralized healthcare system in Tanzania

The wide geographical spread of the Tanzanian population adds a further level of complexity to the logistics of running a national health service as well as a mass treatment programme. It has led to decentralized health and education systems which tend to operate at a district level rather than a central one, in contrast to the countries in the west sub-Saharan region. The distances mean more complicated logistics for drugs and other services to be available in areas far from the capital city.

Within Tanzania, where decentralization has been adopted, each district has a health management team which decides who to treat and which drugs to use. The team oversees both dispensaries and rural health centres, which each usually serve up to 50,000 people and may be manned by a health professional (a qualified nurse) but most likely *not* a medical doctor. If specialized care is needed, patients will be referred to a district or regional hospital. In 2006, Tanzania had just four consultant hospitals, one each for the north, south, east and west areas. As of 2020, Tanzania boasted 337 hospitals.

Despite the relatively high availability of healthcare provision in the country, an estimated two-thirds of the population have problems accessing even primary healthcare, either because they have inadequate funds or because they are unable to travel the not inconsiderable distance to receive treatment. A survey in 2008 showed that there were only two doctors for every 100,000 of the population. More recently, according to a 2012 estimate (2021 update, Global Health Workforce statistics, WHO) there were 0.31 doctors per 10,000 of the population and in 2016 it was 0.14 per 10,000; so the situation has not improved.

Decentralized healthcare model in Uganda

Uganda also has a decentralized health system, a deliberate choice to encourage a sense of ownership among its end-users and, importantly, a sense of responsibility for one's own health. Wide reform across government departments delegated control and resources down to each of the districts and administrative areas were reorganized. In 2007, when we began, there were 81 districts, but by 2020 there were 134 districts plus the city of Kampala. By 2020, Uganda boasted 14 regional, 139 general and 20 private hospitals. It also prided itself on a network of almost 7000 health centres throughout the country, some with theatres and all with qualified medical personnel.

The progress in improving healthcare in Uganda and the implementation of a strategy whereby they successfully educate and create a demand for healthcare amongst the population is nothing short of admirable and could be a splendid example for other governments to follow. This is illustrated in Box 10.1, which details the work of the Vector Control Division, a sub-unit of the Ministry of Health (MoH) in Kampala, in delivering the schistosomiasis/STH control programme for Uganda. SCI was based in this central unit.

In it, the Vector Control Officer, Robert Mulimba, explains that the local population were very aware of NTDs in their community, but before resources came in from SCI, treatment was not forthcoming. He proudly points out that 'when we started the programme there was already a high demand but no medication was available – by publicizing the MoH initiative, the demand was satisfied and 93% coverage was obtained which was higher than elsewhere. Similarly, there was no resistance to taking the pills when treatment arrived.'

Implementation of the SCI programme was rolled out jointly, at the district level, by the District Director of Health Services and District Vector Control Officers (such as Robert). As well as the Ministry of Health, the Ministry of Education was closely involved because of the need to use teachers to deliver the medication to the schoolchildren.

> **Box 10.1. Robert Mulimba on vector control, community engagement and the SCI programme in Busia, Uganda.**
>
> Robert comes from Busia town in the region of the same name. It is located about 300 km east of the capital city, Kampala, on the border between Uganda and Kenya.
> Busia totals 744 km² with a relatively small population of just over 260,000. An estimated 20% are under 5 which sits well with the national average of approximately 50% being under 15 years of age. There are ten sub-counties in Busia and schistosomiasis has been found all over the district. Three sub-counties border Lake Victoria, and in these, schistosomiasis prevalence was 97% in 2002. This has been reduced by annual treatment to an average of 36% as of January 2008. Since that time, integrated NTD control has been implemented in Uganda, but with regular treatment the lower prevalence rate has been maintained. Elimination of schistosomiasis under these highly endemic conditions is not thought to be achievable by the new WHO target of 2030.
> Robert tries to maximize community involvement in health-control measures. In addition to the national- and district-level health centres, they have village health teams – community volunteers who provide information and refer patients. These people are chosen by the community itself, directly planting responsibility amongst local people and ensuring an essential level of inclusion and trust.
> There are also five paid medical doctors in Busia, so one doctor to 52,000 people, and 26 nurses, so 1 nurse to 10,000 people. More doctors and nurses are needed, especially since more people are becoming health-aware and seeking treatment.
> HIV prevalence is higher than the national average (7%) and sits at about 10%. This is mainly due to it being on the Kenyan border and a lot of travellers pass through, going to and from Nairobi. Malaria is still ranked the biggest killer with a prevalence of 43%.

The Failure of Previous Control Projects, 1985–2000

Examples of West African control programmes simply running out of donor funds

In the period 1985–2000, a few of the selected countries did at some stage launch rudimentary schistosomiasis control projects, but they rarely lasted long. They collapsed for a number of reasons. Among these would be a lack of long-term financial commitment for annual treatments, no guaranteed regular supply of praziquantel, inadequate sustainable planning and, usually, a failure to incorporate some level of evaluation to demonstrate success.

For example, a European Union control project was established in Niger in 1991, but was shut down in 1999.

Between 1979 and 1988 in Mali, a schistosomiasis control project funded by GTZ (Gesellschaft für Technische Zusammenarbeit) was set up to focus primarily on irrigation zones and areas with dams such as the Office du Niger and Selingue. (GTZ is the German government technical co-operation agency which encourages sustainable development.) When funding ceased, the Ministry of Health encouraged the continuation of the project by purchasing small amounts of praziquantel each year for hyper-endemic communities. This continued for three years but funds eventually dried up in 1991. Then, between 1996 and 2002, the National Schistosomiasis Control Programme (PNLSH) received some funding from the WHO for targeted control efforts, but not enough to reach national coverage. The WHO funding included research studies on disease prevalence, intensity and distribution in hyper-endemic zones.

And so the Mali government were very excited and relieved in 2003 when the SCI selected Mali as part of its programme, and therefore provided the extra funding needed to buy more praziquantel for expansion, and pay for the training and delivery of the drugs.

Working across West Africa – Mali, Niger and Burkina Faso

Our SCI programmes were launched in Mali, Niger and Burkina Faso between June and October 2003.

Burkina Faso launch

The programme in Burkina Faso prepared by Dr Seydou Touré was accepted for implementation, supported by SCI, and so Howard Thompson and I visited Ouagadougou where we teamed up with Dr Bertrand Sellin of RISEAL, to meet the Minister of Health (Dr Alain Yoda) and finalize an MoU so we could arrange the launch. Unbeknown to us Dr Touré's father was the Prime Minister in Ouagadougou and so this facilitated our entrance in to see the minister. Dr Yoda was, in fact, very amiable and supportive of our proposals to extend treatment to the four kingdoms in Burkina Faso and we visited two of the kings, in Ouagadougou and Ouaigouia.

In Ouagadougou we attended a ceremony which was re-enacted on Friday mornings in the grounds of the King's palace; it depicts the King of Ouagadougou getting very angry when his wife elopes with one of the other kings and he calls for his horse to go and bring back his wife and punish the other king. In the enactment, he is discouraged by all the local dignitaries, and convinced to stay at home and find another wife.

After the ceremony, Howard, Albis,[1] Bertrand and I were invited into the inner sanctuary of the palace and given the chance to explain our plans to offer treatment to all children against schistosomiasis and STH. The king offered us a drink, which we accepted, and his young attendants were sent off to bring four glasses and a bottle of Johnny Walker whisky – at 8 am! His throne was in the middle of a large, rather empty hall, and all the way around the walls were notices saying photographs were forbidden. In his local language the king asked us a favour and when this was translated, I said, 'Of course, what do you want?' It transpired that he wanted a group photo. Once again, he sent his servants away and this time they returned with a camera. He also gave permission for us to use our own cameras.

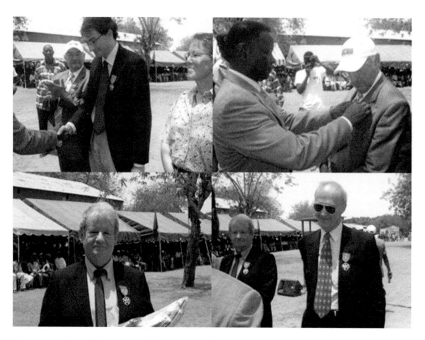

Fig. 10.2. (clockwise) Albis, Alan, Howard and Bertrand receiving the award of Chevalier.

A few days later we visited the second king at Ouaigouia and that was quite a welcome we received. As we walked up the driveway to the palace we were greeted by a dozen men all armed with blunderbusses, which they fired as we went past them. The noise from those guns was ear-splitting and we all jumped every time they were fired. The king was very welcoming (with Coca-Cola, not whisky) and he participated in the treatments we gave at the launch in his city.

The launches in both cities went very well and within a couple of years we had reached national coverage. Our efforts were appreciated, and in 2006, Howard, Albis, Bertrand and I were all presented with a medal by Dr Alain Yoda. We became chevaliers – knights of Burkina Faso. We received a medal, a citation and a small lapel badge. I was wearing this lapel badge at the next World Health Assembly, and descending in the hotel elevator, when a stranger, who turned out to be a Burkina Bey (a man from Burkina Faso), looked at me and asked if what I was wearing was from Burkina Faso. I said 'Yes, I am a chevalier,' and he said 'Wow! I did not know we gave chevaliers to white men.' I smiled sweetly at him and explained how we earned the honour.

Niger launch

On 6 October 2003, the Minister of Health of Niger launched the Schistosomiasis Control Programme of the Government of Niger (Box 10.2). Once again, it was a big affair.

Box 10.2. A typical press release: this one is for the launch in Niger.

On 6 October, the Minister of Health of Niger, Monsieur Mamadou Sourghia, launched the Schistosomiasis Control Programme of the Government of Niger. This ceremony was held at Kollo, a town about 50 kilometers south of Niamey, close to the banks of the Niger River. His audience included hundreds of citizens of Kollo, who are all too familiar with schistosomiasis, and representatives of all levels of government, as well as of WHO, the Institut Pasteur (CERMES), World Food Programme (WFP) and various foreign missions involved in health service delivery in Niger.

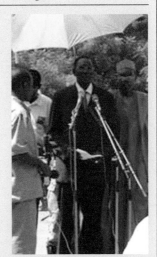

Minister of Health, Mr. Mamadou Sourghia, launches the national control programme

The Governor of Tillaberri Province, where Kollo is located, also gave a speech in which he encouraged the citizens of his region to take advantage of this programme and the medicine which it will make available every year from now on.

Monsieur Sourghia explained that schistosomiasis is second only to malaria in terms of morbidity and social importance in Niger, causing around 3 million people to be seriously infected. He committed the government to a permanent programme of control and urged all those who would be contacted over the coming years by staff of his ministry to respond positively and take advantage of the availability of praziquantel and albendazole tablets which will be freely available.

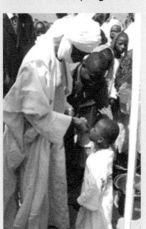

The ministry target was to treat 1 million people by the end of 2004, and twice as many during the course of 2005. They delivered treatment to at least 3 million people by some time in 2006, each person treated being scheduled for a second treatment a year afterwards. Monitoring of the programme was conducted by staff of CERMES (Centre de Recherches Medicales et Scientifiques), which received support from the government of France. Both praziquantel and albendazole were provided by SCI using the Gates Foundation money, along with equipment to support their distribution and to enable surveillance and monitoring activities on an appropriate scale.

Delivery of the programme was through the Ministry of Health's unit PNLBG and was conducted for several years. The results were again very positive and were comparable to the results from Burkina Faso.

Collaboration – SCI is the catalyst

Because Mali, Niger and Burkina Faso are situated on the Niger river basin, the inhabitants living close to the river are at high risk from water-borne diseases such as schistosomiasis, malaria, lymphatic filariasis (LF), guinea worm and onchocerciasis.

SCI set out to assist the health ministry officials who were responsible for parasitic diseases in each of these countries, with the aim of getting them to collaborate with each other, and so stimulate a cost-efficient, integrated approach to the control of schistosomiasis and STH (you may recall that this was the agreement made with our technical committee – that Mali, Niger and Burkina Faso should be considered as an entity, a fourth 'country', to qualify for funding).

Each country had some history of treating one or more NTDs, so brought NTD strengths to the table. Burkina Faso had a strong LF programme, several years old and led by Dr Dominique Kyelem, whereas Mali and Niger were lacking any LF programme and so could benefit from the experience in LF from Dr Kyelem. On the other hand, Mali provided historically strong schistosomiasis research expertise and ultrasound expertise from Dr Moussa Sacko, while Niger had an ongoing trachoma programme which could (and would) be extended into the other two countries. A strong link between the three countries was the presence in each of a French NGO (RISEAL) and a schistosomiasis specialist, Dr Bertrand Sellin, who, with his wife Elizabeth, had spent many years in these countries. (Sadly, Bertrand passed away in 2014.)

As a result, NTD control was expanded into all three countries concurrently, allowing collaborative drug delivery and the development of a standardized M&E programme. The political will in each of these countries was very strong, and each health ministry provided local staff towards the implementation project.

The respective leads of each country's programme ran their own individual schistosomiasis and STH control programmes but ensured that there was genuine collaboration across all; the leads were Dr Seydou Touré in Burkina Faso, Dr Mamadou Traore in Mali and Dr Amadou Garba in Niger. It was so satisfying to work with all of them and see their careers take off. Dr Mamadou Traore went on to join the EU as an expert advisor and Dr Amadou Garba – who quickly mastered English – was later employed by WHO to run their schistosomiasis control programme from Geneva.

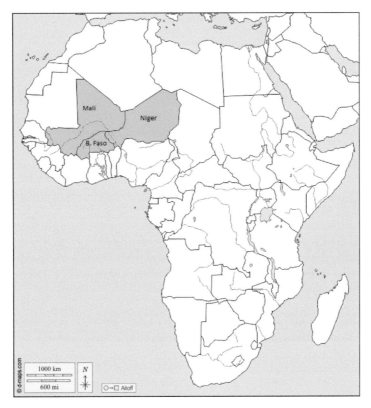

Fig. 10.3. River systems and lakes of Africa highlighting Burkina Faso, Mali and Niger.
(Courtesy of Amadou Garba)

The map of the region (Fig. 10.3) shows the river systems which flow through Niger, Mali and Burkina Faso. Between 1996 and 2006, each country built dams on these systems, for power, reservoirs and irrigation schemes. The 'favorable conditions for snails and for increased water contact' (Garba *et al.*, 2006) led, inevitably, to increases in schistosomiasis.

Tiered training systems and workshops in Mali and Niger

The West Africans knew what needed to be done. In Mali, the training and development of local staff was conducted by the local control team (PNLSH) employing a tiered training system. Prior to each mass treatment campaign, training workshops were conducted to ensure all health and education officials, drug distributors, supervisors and teachers had a strong understanding of the treatment campaign goals. They learned about the appropriate treatment strategies, the selected treatment tools and how to manage possible side-effects.

A similar training system was put in place in Niger. In 2004, a national-level 'training of trainers' (ToT) workshop was conducted. The national co-ordinator from the Ministry of Health for the schistosomiasis and STH control programme (PNLBG) and the deputy co-ordinator conducted the training. They addressed senior staff from the division of disease control and from the health ministry's division of school health in order that they could conduct further ToT sessions. The ToT workshops were conducted in each region and district and repeated prior to each campaign.

The workshops reviewed the transmission cycle of both schistosomiasis and STH as well as topics covering aspects of MDAs. For example, they described the benefits of both praziquantel and albendazole and how to use the WHO praziquantel dose pole to administer an appropriate measure of praziquantel. They also detailed the procedures for managing possible severe adverse effects, noting what to look for when conducting MDA supervision. And they were shown how to train district-level health and education officials to carry out similar work.

In this way knowledge was cascaded down through local-level training workshops to prepare teachers, community drug distributors and local health agents. Overall, the local-level training workshops focused on how to treat the target communities, not on the transmission cycle of both parasites or the pharmacokinetics of the drugs.

The Ministry of Health programme in Mali was also well received and the launch was attended by the First Lady of Mali who treated the first school girl. The event was very colourful and well attended by dignitaries and diplomats.

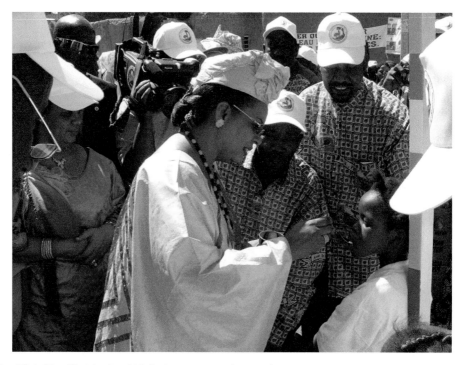

Fig. 10.4. The First Lady of Mali gives out praziquantel.

Effectiveness of campaigns in Burkina Faso

The Burkina Faso national programme used nurses, teachers and community volunteers to deliver the tablets, but still achieved a full national coverage of treatment in 2005. In some villages we targeted children in schools and, by visiting the communities, reached out to school-age children who were not attending school. As a result, we could report that the campaign provided treatment to over 3.3 million school-age children, representing 90.8% of the estimated school-age children in the country (Gabrielli *et al.*, 2006).

Significantly, the in-country cost of delivery was less than 10 US cents per treatment, and the cost including drugs was a mere 32 US cents per treatment. Costs are difficult to standardize because different countries have different needs in terms of what they pay per diem or for local fuel and training. The cost of praziquantel before the donation started was standard at 20 US cents, on average, per child, the equivalent of 2.5 tablets at 8 cents each.

In order to evaluate the effectiveness of each of the various SCI-supported campaigns in terms of reduced prevalence and reduced intensity of infection, a sample of the school-age children were examined prior to treatment (i.e. at baseline) and at both one year and two years after receiving praziquantel. The global average with all praziquantel-based MDAs, after one treatment, results in a significantly reduced overall prevalence. In this particular cohort study – 1727 children (Touré *et al.*, 2008) (Figure 10.5) – the results were even better, with prevalence in children reduced from 59.6% prior to treatment to 6.2% after one year. This level of prevalence was maintained after two years, with levels only increasing marginally to 7.7%.

Effectively, infection levels had dropped by an overall 87.1% across two years, from which we knew that blood in the urine would have disappeared, and could presume that these children would not suffer again in the future.

Similarly, this picture was mirrored by the drop in intensity of infection, which is a measure of the number of eggs present in an infected individual. Intensity was significantly reduced from 94.2 eggs/10 ml urine prior to treatment to only 1.0 eggs/10 ml at one year post-treatment, and 6.8 eggs/10 ml after two years, an overall reduction of 92.8%.

Importantly, before treatment, 25% of school children examined were heavily infected and passing over 50 eggs/10 ml urine, and this percentage decreased to only 0.4% at one year post-treatment and remained below 2% at two years post-treatment. Again, these reductions suggest that the children have been protected from organ damage in the future.

In addition to the cohort follow-up, at the two-year post-treatment point, researchers also conducted a cross-sectional survey on 7- to 14-year olds from the same schools but who were outside the original cohort (Fig. 10.5). The additional data indicated a significant 77% reduction in prevalence and an equally significant 80% reduction in intensity of infection, compared to

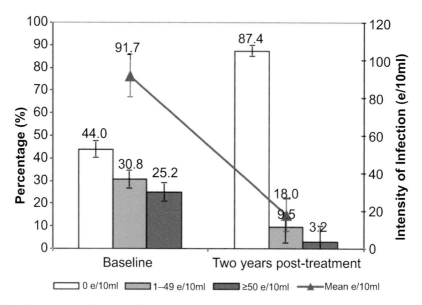

Fig. 10.5. Proportion of light and heavy infections in the schoolchildren outside the study cohort before and two years after treatment. The line represents the arithmetic mean intensity of infection (Touré *et al.*, 2008).

levels prior to treatment. The proportion of heavy *S. haematobium* infections in children was similarly reduced from over 25% to 3.2% two years after treatment.

Work in East Africa – Tanzania, Uganda and Zambia

Key factors to the successful roll-out of a major national health-based programme will include the challenges offered by the geography over which it must occur and the political backdrop against which it must operate.

Geographical landscape

Tanzania is home to Mount Kilimanjaro, almost 6000 square miles of Serengeti plains, the Ngorongoro Crater, several game parks, and the spice farms and coconut-palmed beaches of Zanzibar. Tanzania is widely known for its enduring appeal to tourists worldwide. Indeed, after agriculture, which accounts for 80% of the country's GDP, tourism to the game parks is an important and growing sector of the economy. Uganda tourism has increased, with

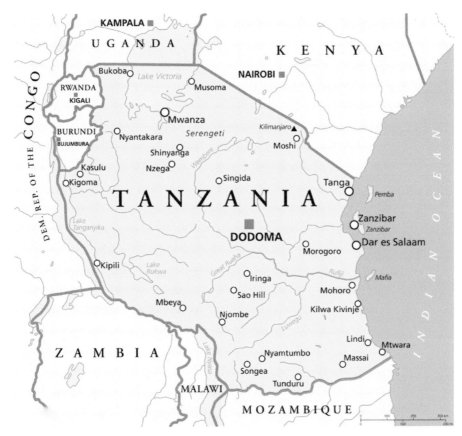

Fig. 10.6. Tanzania showing main tourist features, towns and lakes. (Based on www. africaguide.com)

naturalists visiting the beautiful Kisinga Channel between lakes Albert and George, the Murchison Falls and the Queen Elizabeth Game Park. Uganda tourism has recovered from a low during Idi Amin's period as president.

Zambia also boasts well-stocked game parks, and tourists visit the beautiful Lake Kariba and gain access to the Victoria Falls which separates Zambia and Zimbabwe. But despite their stunning and dramatic landscapes, outside of the capital cities and these tourist destinations, the heartlands of these three countries house a rural population mired in poverty and diseases; something that is rarely seen in the big cities and by the many healthy and wealthy foreign visitors.

There are no half-measures in Tanzania. If it's a mountain then it's the highest, if it's a crater then it's the widest, and if it's a lake it's the largest (Lake Victoria is the largest lake in Africa and the second largest freshwater lake in the world). In fact, Tanzania as a whole has an abundance of inland fresh water with lakes dotted around the Great Rift Valley which runs through the heart of the country. Lake Tanganyika is Africa's longest and deepest, and together with Rukwa and Nyasa, they are all located on the western branch of the valley, while lakes Natron, Manyara and Eyasi shelter around the eastern side of the country.

The Great Lakes: home to the people of the region

There is no shortage of fresh water in the three eastern countries. The lakes in all of them provide the life force for communities who live around them and indeed for many who live further away. Also, in Uganda, the banks of the river Nile – which runs north from its source at Jinja on Lake Victoria – provide all-year water for the inhabitants. The shores of Lake Victoria, which border Uganda, Kenya and Tanzania, support one of the most densely populated regions in the world.

Fishing provides the local people with their livelihood, and the waters irrigate the fertile land. But these bountiful fresh waters have a dark side; they harbour the intermediate hosts of parasites which cause malaria, LF, schistosomiasis and river blindness.

Political landscape

Whereas Tanzania has had a relatively peaceful political life thanks to Mwalimu Julius Nyerere, the first president, Uganda has suffered frequent political strife. Fortunately, after a troubled political period under Idi Amin (1971–1979), and even President Obote (1979–1986), President Museveni (since 1986) has brought stability to the country and is now President for life. Yet even during his rule there have been pockets of unrest, especially in the northern Ugandan territories with the Lord's Resistance Army (LRA) and the militia which have periodically attacked from neighbouring Congo and Sudan. However, the country has, so far, battled to overcome these threats.

The political landscape in Zambia has remained relatively stable, in particular when compared to regional neighbours. After independence in 1964, President Kenneth Kaunda ruled until 1991. Zambia has had several presidents since then, two of whom died in office. Since 1991, though, when multi-party elections were introduced, Zambia has enjoyed relative political stability, and the transition of power between parties has occurred smoothly. The current president is Edgar Lungu, who was elected in 2016.

A rather ugly incident during roll-out in Tanzania

The success of programmes like SCI rely on the good will and engagement of the local population and it is therefore vitally important that such programmes are received as good news. Unfortunately, bad publicity can very quickly and substantially undermine an otherwise good cause. There was a time, in 2005, when we perhaps became complacent about publicity and in particular about preparing communities for the MDA, which gave rise to bad press and a misrepresentation, which, in turn, precipitated anger, confusion and a dangerous reaction. The SCI was launched nationally in Dodoma, Tanzania, that year. Schoolchildren were given praziquantel and albendazole (for STHs) in 65 districts drawn from 11 endemic regions of the country, including Tabora. It was in three schools near Morogoro that our incident occurred.

Twenty-nine children developed short-term, adverse side-effects (headache and stomach pains) after receiving the drugs and were admitted to hospital. After a thorough investigation, it was concluded that parents and children had failed to be provided with sufficient information on how to prepare for treatment and deal with any side-effects, with the result that children and their parents panicked.

Bad news travels fast and easily escalates to inflated and misleading proportions. A number of confusing statements incited fear in the community. A Tanzanian national newspaper, *The Guardian*, reported that parents had threatened violence towards teachers after some schoolchildren had 'developed breathing difficulties and became unconscious after swallowing the medicine, while others developed serious muscle convulsions and swollen faces'. Where the journalist received his information we are still not sure. We quickly commissioned an official investigation from Dar es Salaam and the results of the investigation showed that the children actually experienced headache, dizziness, body weakness, abdominal discomfort and vomiting. These are not unexpected side-effects and are very similar to the list found on most drug-prescribing information inserts, but they are also very rare. In this case there appeared to have been a knock-on effect with children who were actually not ill mirroring the side-effects of the first true casualty.

Incorrect dosing and poor quality of praziquantel were put forward as possible causes. These were, however, dismissed as the reason for the side-effects, so investigations turned towards implementation events leading up to, during and after the treatment day. The investigators found that most children who experienced the adverse events had not received adequate food before, during and after drug intake. They also concluded that the implementation process at the district level had suffered from poor advocacy caused either by insufficient funds and/or complacency and low participation by members of the Regional Health Management Team and District Health Management teams. So even though we had felt that sensitization and awareness had been effective at the regional and district levels, this information had not trickled through to community leaders and stakeholders, leaving parents unprepared, and teachers not aware of the need to provide some nourishment before the pills were swallowed.

The sequence of events had been further complicated by the local and parliamentary elections, which had been delayed, causing them to coincide with the treatment days. Political events were absorbing the district authority's time and resources, diverting attention away from the health campaign. At the same time, the country's doctors were on strike and district medical officers were asked to cover for them rather than attend the SCI campaign preparation activities.

Our conclusion was that the pre-treatment dissemination of information about the children needing to have eaten *prior to treatment*, and the delivery of a warning of possible side-effects was sadly inadequate in these particular village schools.

Reports in the media inevitably gave rise to a flurry of rumours which spread around the community casting doubt on the programme. The sequence of events had the potential to seriously damage the Tanzanian effort had the SCI advocacy programme not buffered and quelled the adversity.

Important lessons were learned from this isolated incident and in every country since, communication of information to local people has been stepped up. The ministries of health and education in Tanzania issued press releases and efforts were made through the media to allay fear and mistrust by informing the public that the programme 'will improve their health, not damage it'. Future campaigns also disseminated the message that 'this was not family planning but a de-worming exercise'. Eventually, the media campaign was well received and, after a break of two years, the SCI assistance to Tanzania was reinstated, with parents and schoolchildren returning for treatment.

One very serious and scary aspect of this incident was that an SCI staff member and a social science researcher from Birkbeck College were present in the same village at the time, and they felt very threatened by the local population who became quite belligerent. The outcome was that the supervisors of the researcher (Professors Tim Allen and Melissa Parker) were very vocal in their criticism of the SCI for several years afterwards. Their criticism was understandable and ensured that we never made the same mistake again.

The Need to Publicize

Communities see the benefits first-hand

The hope was that as the SCI outreach and coverage expanded, the benefits of treatment would be noticed. As infection rates fell, fewer children would suffer debilitation by the disease and the communities would witness their children's growth and realize the benefits of taking treatment first-hand.

It was therefore important for SCI to analyse and publish the programme results in scientific journals and for those results to be disseminated to ministers of health from these and other countries. Careful M&E would be needed to provide evidence of the benefits of wide-scale treatment to different interested parties. These included showing national governments in endemic countries the achievements of their neighbours so they would respond positively to future offers of support for their programmes. Results also needed to be publicized so that international donor countries, foundations and pharmaceutical companies, would continue and hopefully expand their donations.

The M&E involved annually examining a cohort of children and measuring their progressive response to the treatment over several years (see Chapter 14). For the first time in sub-Saharan Africa, SCI provided evidence that in most of the *S. haematobium* endemic areas, praziquantel treatment, on a large scale once every year, significantly reduced prevalence and the intensity of schistosomiasis (as measured by a reduction in eggs and the absence of blood in the urine). To a lesser extent, the M&E showed that parallel albendazole treatment reduced the prevalence of STHs.

However, we also showed that in some foci (now termed 'hot spots') eggs were still being produced; and so in these areas we needed to provide more frequent treatment to maintain acceptably low levels. The hot spots were usually close to recognizable water bodies and snail-breeding sites where there was contact by adults and children.

Our ultimate aim was that, as a result of five years of treatment and a positive M&E, the number of rural populations needing regular treatment could be reduced to more easily manageable levels. The local health services with their limited resources then might become more ready, willing and able to meet the local treatment costs.

When this was achieved, the SCI could consider scaling down its technical assistance and financial support and achieve its goal of handing over a sustainable, cost-effective control programme to a government-led national campaign within countries.

Note

[1] Albis Gabrielli is a medical doctor who joined SCI as a French speaker to oversee our early programmes in Burkina Faso, Mali and Niger. After a most successful period at SCI he was headhunted to join the World Health Organization in their Neglected Tropical Diseases section.

11 Schistosomiasis – Mapping the Disease

For governments in Africa, faced with a high percentage of their population infected with treatable NTDs, mass treatment programmes present a daunting task and great expense. Control of onchocerciasis and lymphatic filariasis (LF) requires the annual treatment of every individual in the endemic area using the medication ivermectin for onchocerciasis, and ivermectin and albendazole in combination to treat LF.

MDAs and Survey Mapping

To implement a control programme cost-effectively, SCI needed to arrange and fund a mapping of schistosomiasis throughout each of the countries to create a record of the spatial distribution of the disease and associated factors. This was achieved by MoH-trained staff who would sample cohorts of schoolchildren from a selection of schools across the countries by testing urine and stool samples for parasite eggs. In this way the districts in need of treatment were identified and, in particular, focal pockets of intense disease were highlighted. Armed with prevalence and intensity of infection data, control programmes could then be designed, budgeted for, planned and administered, with districts qualifying for treatment included in the exercise.

This chapter discusses the techniques used to map, how we used these to successfully deliver our MDA programmes in Uganda and reduce disease prevalence, and considers how acceptability of MDA grew with such success.

What Factors are Mapped?

Parasitic diseases (the NTDs) are dependent on the local demography, the presence of water bodies and the distribution of the vectors, and are therefore focal in distribution.

The factors which determine the presence or absence of vector snails include temperature, rainfall, water body type, water velocity and altitude – all of which have an effect on the distribution of the snail hosts and therefore on the schistosomiasis transmission. Other factors that are mapped will include the prevalence of the parasite in the local population. For example, in some parts of coastal East Africa the temperatures are too high for the snail host *Biomphalaria* species, which explains the absence of *S. mansoni* in this region, while the *Bulinus* species are in their element and so *S. haematobium* is prevalent in the coastal regions. Away from the coast, *S. mansoni* may thrive, but then at higher altitudes the cooler conditions may prevent development of the parasite in the snail. Hence the focal distribution of the intermediate host snails and the two schistosome species.

Snails versus Habitats versus Infection (Modelling)

Mathematical model parameters used in the mapping of *S. haematobium* and *S. mansoni* include the known biology and distribution of the specific freshwater snails which are the intermediate hosts for schistosomes.

Thus, in rural Uganda, the concentration of *Biomphalaria* snail hosts in the lakeshores and the extensive human/water contact explains the very high prevalence of *S. mansoni* and the high morbidity there; and, equally, their absence explains the lower prevalence away from the lakeshores.

In contrast, *S. haematobium* is hardly ever prevalent in Ugandan villages, because *Bulinus* snails are not found in Uganda. However, in the coastal area of Tanzania, there are three *Bulinus* host species: *B. nasutus*, *B. africanus* and *B. globosus*, which occupy a mosaic of habitats such that transmission is widespread. (These important results were published before Tanganyika became Tanzania, when Lake Victoria was referred to as Lake Province (Webbe, 1962).)

Both species of the parasite are endemic in Tanzania but are found focally in areas which suit their own snail host. *S. haematobium* is widespread within every district to some extent but is concentrated down the coastline. The *S. mansoni* infection is known to be endemic primarily around Lake Victoria, although there have been infections reported in and around Arusha and Moshi in northern Tanzania.

Strangely, when we turn to Lake Malawi, which borders Tanzania, for some reason the *Bulinus* snails are more prevalent, leading to a high risk of *S. haematobium*. But Lake Malawi has an epidemiological story of its own because recent fishing activity intensified there, leading to a much-reduced density of fish, which in turn has allowed the snail population to increase. Hence there has been a sharp increase in the risk of schistosomiasis. This hypothesis seems to be supported by the high number of UK tourists who, after snorkelling in Lake Malawi, return home with blood in their urine caused by an *S. haematobium* infection.

Diagnostic Techniques to Determine Disease Prevalence

The diagnostic techniques used in mapping vary with species. For the diagnosis of *S. mansoni* we had no alternative in 2003 but to using egg detection in stool samples, which involves the rather unpleasant technique of collecting stool samples and then examining them microscopically to count the number of eggs. The samples were examined using a technique referred to as the 'Kato-Katz' method, which allows for a calculation of a quantitative estimate of the number of eggs per gram of faeces. A small quantity (40 mg) of stool is pushed through a sieve which has a mesh size just larger than the size of the schistosome eggs (160 microns) and so the eggs pass through but larger particles are left behind. A measured quantity of the sieved faeces is then gently squashed onto a glass microscope slide under a coverslip and the eggs are counted in this given sample under a microscope.

This microscopic method provides a definitive diagnosis and an estimation of *S. mansoni* prevalence and intensity (more eggs are assumed to mean more worms).

It should be pointed out that the method relies on the examination of only a tiny sample of faeces and is therefore insensitive for people with light infections.

Today, an easier and more sensitive dipstick-in-urine test has been developed for detecting *S. mansoni* – with proven success. The dipstick has antibodies which respond to the eggs excreted in the urine – no stool samples need be examined! The test is more sensitive than the Kato-Katz, is a lot quicker and, as you can imagine, more pleasant to carry out – and is specific to *S. mansoni*.

For *S. haematobium* our first diagnostic is the easily identifiable symptom of blood in the urine and the prevalence of this species can be crudely mapped using a 'blood-in-urine' questionnaire. This is a particularly useful and proven tool for surveying school-age children in high endemic areas. A more sensitive and accurate quantitative estimate of the number of *S. haematobium* parasites present is determined by filtering 10 ml of urine sample through microscopic gauze, which traps the eggs, and then counting the eggs under a microscope. For mapping purposes, and for deciding whether to treat or not, the questionnaire is quick and simple, but for accurate scientific monitoring the microscope methods are required.

The blood-in-urine questionnaire provided a national picture of *S. haematobium* infection risk in Tanzania after teachers in over 11,000 schools answered our request for data, and these results were then corroborated by examining a smaller sample of urine samples in the key areas. The results of this parasitology survey were used to construct regional distribution and prevalence maps as shown in the Fig. 11.1.

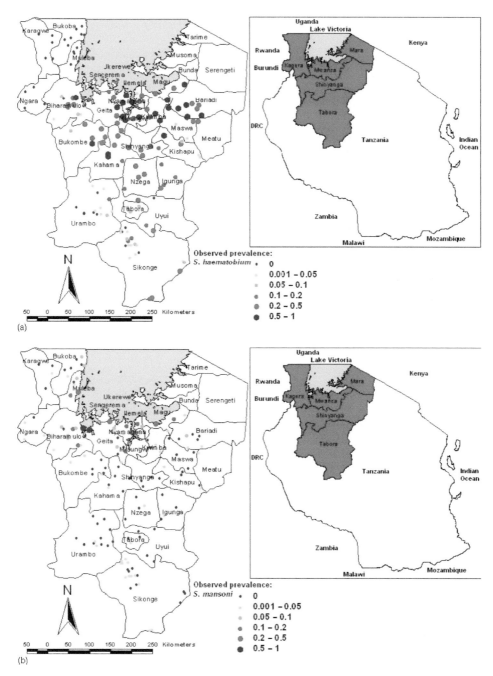

Fig. 11.1. Geographical distribution of schools surveyed in north-west Tanzania and prevalence of (a) *S. haematobium* and (b) *S. mansoni*. (From Clements *et al.*, 2006.)

Mapping to an Administrative Unit in a Country

The design of our mapping exercise has to provide us with enough information to make a treatment decision at the appropriate 'implementation unit' level considering the focal nature of the disease. In Tanzania, for example, the optimum unit has been determined to be the relatively small administration unit known as a 'ward'. Once the prevalence in each ward has been estimated, the WHO guidelines are consulted and applied to determine the level of treatment to be implemented throughout that ward.

For every district targeted for treatment, a colour-coded map was developed showing prevalence in each ward, and from that data a treatment plan was developed according to WHO guidelines (see Fig. 11.2).

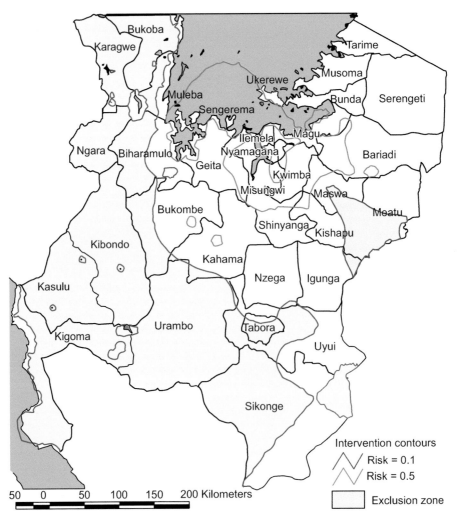

Fig. 11.2. Intervention map for north-west Tanzania with prevalence contours defining areas for treatment. (From Clements *et al.*, 2006.)

In Tanzania, the maps were originally created using the questionnaire data only – i.e. showing levels of *S. haematobium* infection. These maps were then overlaid with results from the *S. mansoni* parasitological mapping. The prevalence levels of any wards were then accurately colour-coded to reflect the highest level of either infection. For example, any wards bordering the lake shore initially had a <10% risk level because *S. haematobium* infection was low in that area, however, *S. mansoni* infection was over 50% so the map was changed to colour those wards red to indicate the need for annual treatment at the community level.

In West Africa, the prevalence of both schistosomiasis and STH also shows a marked focal distribution. In some districts in Niger, with many permanent and semi-permanent ponds and rivers, a large proportion of the local population was infected and so they were targeted by the Programme Nationale Lutte Bilharzia (PNLBG) through community-based treatment. In other districts, such as those in the northern part of the country, only a few villages indicated a high prevalence, justifying community-based treatment, and elsewhere we concentrated on reaching school-age children.

Occasionally, prevalence by village varied from under 5% to over 80% even within one district so collecting enough data and looking at the smaller administrative level is essential to avoid cases of over-treatment or under-treatment.

New Technologies (GIS Overlays)

In recent years, more sophisticated tools and techniques have been developed and validated, and these have enabled epidemiologists to develop maps to a higher specification incorporating more detailed data. In Uganda and Tanzania, geographical information systems (GIS) have been used to map the distribution of infection as well as to overlay environmental information with ecological data on the preferred habitats of the parasites.

Upon analysis of GIS results from Uganda, the hypothesis prediction that prevalence of infection was highest nearest the lake shore and along rivers was confirmed to be true. The effect of high altitude was shown to limit transmission and it indicated that there was no transmission above 1400 m and if total annual rainfall was less than 900 mm. In a later stage, using high-resolution satellite-generated data to define lakes and rivers, it was found that prevalence consistently exceeded 50% in areas within 5 km of lakes Victoria, Kyoga, Albert and the Albert Nile. These findings have helped those implementing the national treatment programmes to not only identify where it is least likely to find *S. mansoni*, but also where infection and impact on the community is likely to be greatest. This means that those people most at risk could be prioritized for treatment and resources allocated accordingly to maximum effect.

At-risk Populations – Disease Prevalence Estimates Post-mapping

In most African countries, almost half of the population is aged under 15 with most of the remainder under 65 – and Tanzania and Uganda are no exception. This means that only half of the population are in the economically productive age band of 15–64. It also means that a large percentage of the total population are of school age, which is when many infectious diseases, particularly parasitic, are most likely to reach maximum prevalence. Relative to other countries in the group selected for support by the SCI, Tanzania is the largest and is inhabited by a largely rural population. In 2003, approximately 80% of Tanzanians lived in rural environments where the median time to a water source was 27 minutes. Only 1.6% of homes had access to electricity and 54% were without access to improved sanitation. The situation has changed very significantly, and by 2020 over 78% of the population had access to grid electricity.

SCI Reduces Prevalence in Uganda but Hotspots Remain

In 2002, at the time when the Ugandan Ministry of Health submitted its application for SCI support, schistosomiasis in the country's endemic regions was almost exclusively due to *S. mansoni*. This intestinal form of the disease was found in 38 out of 56 districts whilst *S. haematobium* was found in only two districts. We had estimated that approximately 1.7 million people were infected with schistosomiasis, representing 7.8% of the population, with 13% projected to be at risk. However, following the mapping exercise conducted in 2003, this estimate rose to 4 million infected (14%) and 16.7 million at risk.

Because of the focal nature of schistosomiasis, it is, however, meaningless to quote a national percentage and to target a percentage nationwide; it is better to report and target to reduce the prevalence to less than 10% in every sub-district.

After years of SCI support, most sub-counties had reduced the prevalence to below 10%, and some reached as low as 5%, although some sub-counties – which we have labelled 'hotspots' – achieved only marginal reduction despite annual treatment from 2002 to 2007. It is difficult to understand why these hot spots exist when treatments have been delivered regularly, but we assume it is because they are villages situated close to lakes Albert and Victoria. These villages show a high intensity of transmission, and so it is likely that villagers are re-infected almost immediately after treatment. To combat the disease levels in these hot spots we offer the residents of these villages two treatments every year.

2010: Offering Treatment to Inhabitants of the Ugandan Islands Situated in Lake Victoria

One special situation had been put on hold when we first started our programme, namely the fishing communities of the myriad small islands in the

Ugandan section of Lake Victoria. These people presented us with significant logistical difficulty and were initially prohibitively expensive to reach, so could not be included in the first rounds of the treatment programme. However, we addressed this in 2010 when we successfully expanded our scope of treatment to bring these missing people into our programme.

Improving Economics to Maintain Ugandan Success

Notwithstanding the success of the Ugandan Ministry of Health in reducing prevalence to below 5% in many sub-counties, these levels will only be maintained, first, with a maintenance programme of continued annual treatment and, second, when the basic standard of living is raised across rural regions, with clean water provided and sanitation levels improved. Even by 2016 the coverage with electricity was only 60% in urban areas and 26% in rural Uganda.

The more stable political background in Uganda is helping to drive forward change and the government has committed to economic improvement which means delivering electricity to as many homes across the country as possible. However, Uganda also requires improved health education, promoted using local media. Then, as local understanding of health needs improves, the people will be encouraged to filter water or even to boil and purify it for washing and drinking rather than using dirty and contaminated water from the lakes. As an aside, the Ugandan Director General of Health was quoted as saying that in his opinion, the availability of electricity would result in huge changes in people's lifestyles, leading to a different work ethic and more social life after sunset.

A Typical SCI Visit in Uganda – Painting a Picture of Advocacy, Training and Implementation

The role of district health officers

Our pre-treatment training was aimed at district health officers and their assistants and teachers, and the main messages were to ensure the targeted population had taken some food, and then to tell the difference between albendazole (one tablet for each person) and praziquantel (dose by dose pole), usually two or three for children and four or five for adults. Additionally, they were shown how to determine the dose each individual needed by standing each person against the dose pole, with their shoes off, hats off, babies off their backs and generally one person at a time. The aim was to deliver approximately 40 mg/kg to everyone – one tablet for every 15 kg in weight. By ensuring that local personnel are trained and understand the importance of their roles, continued high standards are more likely in the long run.

Village meeting to explain the importance of the treatment

A week or so before the designated day that praziquantel is handed out, the district vector control officer (let's call him Simpa) and his team make sure that as many people as possible know about the planned activity on the treatment day. All residents in each village are urged to attend a talk on the reasons why treatment is important and how it can benefit their lives. 'Sensitisation', as it is known locally, is essential because district officers need to explain not only the benefits to people but also the possible mild side-effects, before anyone can be expected just to swallow free medicines. The sensitization aims to prevent any misconceptions about what is being offered and prevent any innate suspicion which may be unjustifiably associated with the treatment programme (lesson learned from the 'ugly incident in Tanzania').

Everyone needs to be aware of the possible side-effects to alleviate worry if some do occur. It is important that as many people as possible turn up on the treatment day to ensure maximum coverage and compliance. Simpa explains how this simple and safe treatment kills any worms currently inside the children and, in doing so, prevents future damage to their livers, intestines and bladders.

At the meeting, the local village health and education officers describe how children are likely to have been infected with schistosomiasis (bilharzia) and stress that because of the absence of clean water supplies and latrines, these worms can survive and re-infect the whole community. The message they try to get across is that until more permanent improvements to the environment are made, the community should understand how they get infected and try, where possible, to modify their behaviour; and avoid relieving themselves in places which lead to their excreta reaching lakes and rivers. Sadly, it will take time for many rural communities in sub-Saharan Africa to be provided with adequate supplies of clean running water and/or latrines, and so taking a curative dose of praziquantel every year currently represents the best available practical option for better health, both immediately and in the longer term. These immediate benefits are huge in terms of better energy, but they may not be long-lasting if people get re-infected quickly.

For almost everyone, the concept of a parasite living in a human body but then infecting a snail as an essential part of the life cycle is difficult to fathom and understand. Even the fact that the parasite larvae leave snails and swim in fresh water is hard to understand, but for this parasite to then enter through unbroken human skin, and survive as it passes through the lungs to the liver, to meet a lifelong worm sexual partner, is even more difficult to believe. If we can convince people of this life cycle, they will understand the need for better hygiene and care to avoid unnecessary water contact.

The health officers also need to explain why annual treatments are necessary and to stress that while praziquantel kills adult worms, it does not kill the immature worms which may be in the body, nor does it offer protection from future infection.

One other drawback to praziquantel is that the tablets themselves are relatively large and their taste is very unpleasant, so the younger children need to be watched carefully to ensure the tablets are swallowed and not chewed and spat out. The unpleasant taste is a deterrent for reaching the optimal coverage, and although praziquantel has no serious adverse effects, many children suffer some level of stomach pains and any episodes of vomiting can quickly reduce compliance in a campaign. Overall, though, its toxicity is low (Frohberg, 1984) and those side-effects observed tend to be mild and transient (Berhe *et al.*, 1999).

The worst side-effect seems to be the vomiting and/or stomach pains, which are probably due to chemicals released from dying schistosomes (Cioli and Pica-Mattoccia, 2003), so again are probably linked to the intensity of infection or the number of dead worms present in the person treated (Polderman *et al.*, 1984; Olds *et al.*, 1999).

Treatment is less likely to cause discomfort and is better absorbed if the tablets are taken after food and not on an empty stomach; so wherever possible, SCI encourages schools to try to provide some breakfast of porridge, or at least some light food such as biscuits or rice, for all children to take before treatment.

And now for the treatment day

It was the last day of the school term and the lakeside fishing village in Mukono district in Uganda was buzzing with playful giggling and wide-eyed curiosity as we drove up. Children as young as 4 carried their baby siblings on their backs whilst others found our bulky 4x4 vehicle a fitting substitute for a climbing-frame when our backs were turned. Older men, mainly fishermen, were dragged out from their huts to show the *wazungu* (white men) their swollen legs, symptomatic of LF; another vector-borne disease common in parts of sub-Saharan Africa. Women were nowhere to be seen.

Together with the village chief, Simpa, who is Mukono's District Vector Control Officer, sets up our makeshift treatment station under the shelter of a mango tree a stone's throw from the water's edge; the same water that was the source of the village's livelihood yet equally the source of so much disease. He sits at the desk and the tree's broad leaves offer him some respite from the punishing heat of the midday sun. The village lies approximately one mile south of the equator and with the sun directly overhead, little can escape its piercing and unforgiving rays. Yet for roughly eight months of the year, it rains heavily early in the day, giving rise to the abundant lush green vegetation so typical of the region.

We did not need much in the way of equipment – mass drug administration is not rocket science. We brought out our dose poles (vertical poles marked off in 'tablets' rather than metres) and set up posters to explain the MDA. Two large white plastic containers are placed in front of Simpa sitting at the desk with the registry: one has praziquantel typed in large letters across it, the other is full of albendazole tablets – drugs for schistosomiasis and STH, respectively.

The community slowly but surely comes out and gathers round to be measured and receive the appropriate number of praziquantel tablets for their height. Water is handed out with the tablets to wash them down.

Health Messages in School Curriculum are Key

In our East African countries, much of the improvement in healthcare can be related to changes to the national school curriculum which have incorporated essential health messages. These schemes recognize that health education, including hygiene and behavioural changes, significantly reduce illness. The same is true of control of schistosomiasis and other NTDs. A pivotal feature of the SCI programme has been to train teachers to relay the message that everyone is ultimately responsible for their own health and well-being.

Most health messages which emanate from a government-driven school curriculum tend to focus on HIV and safe sex. These messages, literally, became clear upon visiting a school near Lake Victoria; on the exterior walls were stencilled, in large bold lettering:

- Delay sex
- Be kind and helpful
- Avoid bad touches
- Stay at school

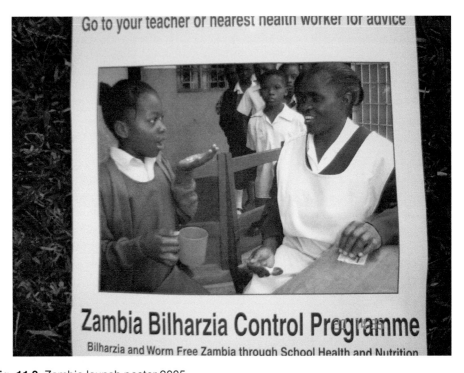

Fig. 11.3. Zambia launch poster 2005.

Box 11.1. Burkina Faso integrates NTD programmes.

Dr Seydou Touré, a medical doctor, was for eight years the SCI national co-ordinator for Burkina Faso

Dr Seydou Touré was employed by the Burkina Faso Ministry of Health. In 2002, when SCI offered money to the country, he was appointed to the position of national co-ordinator for schistosomiasis and STH control. He has seen the national schistosomiasis control programme through from scratch to today's successful programme which has delivered well over 5 million treatments.

'When I started work on schistosomiasis and STHs, we had no control programme so I had to conduct surveys and collect data. Our national health plan addressed NTDs on paper but there wasn't any money to fund wide-scale implementation,' explained Touré.

Other NTDs such as lymphatic filariasis, guinea worm, as well as HIV, malaria, leprosy amongst others had national programmes, but because the price of praziquantel was so high during the nineties, nothing had been done about schistosomiasis.

Burkino Faso is among the world's 50 poorest countries with an average income of $400 per capita, which is about half the average income for sub-Saharan Africa. Its inhabitants are the poorest of the poor. However, the country has a history of research on schistosomiasis dating back to 1956 and the work of the Institute Pasteur. Further work was carried out during the 1980s.

Touré conducted a survey in 2004 to determine the distribution of disease throughout the three climatic zones found in Burkina Faso. Urinary schistosomiasis was found everywhere but more in the Saharan and less in the Sudanian zone, whilst intestinal disease was mainly found in the Sudanian zone.

In 2004, the SCI assisted Burkina Faso to launch a control programme in hyper-endemic regions treating one million school-age children. By 2005, 2.5 million children were treated in the endemic Saharian zone. In 2006, children were retreated in the hyper-endemic zone. By the close of 2008, four mass drug administrations (MDAs) had been completed, with most children having been treated twice.

As a result of new funding from the American government (USAID), Burkino Faso implemented 'integrated control' moving schistosomiasis MDAs into a combined treatment programme for several NTDs. 'We want to integrate schistosomiasis and STH control with lymphatic filariasis, onchocerciasis and trachoma. It would actually be more beneficial to integrate and treat all,' stated Dr Seydou. For four years Burkina Faso used a combination of SCI funds and USAID funds to achieve national coverage.

In 2007, the ministry of health recognized the achievement by awarding a Chevalier medal to each of Professor Alan Fenwick, Director of SCI, Mr Howard Thompson, Deputy Director of SCI, Dr Albis Gabrielli, SCI programme manager and the late Dr Bertrand Sellin, Director of RISEAL, a collaborating NGO.

In 2011 the USAID changed their funding policy and the successful NTD control programme was taken over through another NGO HKI where it continues to this day.

12 Drugs – Mobilizing the African Marketplace to Paralyse the Worm

Once swallowed, praziquantel is absorbed into the individual's blood stream and the circulating praziquantel then begins a sequence of powerful effects on any schistosome worms in the blood. Strangely, for a drug that has been used for 50 years, the exact mode of action is not entirely known although there is some experimental evidence that it increases the permeability of the membranes of the parasite's cells for calcium ions. This increases the electrical potential between the inside and outside of the cells, which induces parasite cell contraction, resulting in paralysis of the worm.

What is certain is that the worms do lose their grip inside the blood vessels and, dislodged from their site of habitation, they are flushed through the body to be destroyed by the host's immune reaction.

This chapter expands on the story of a unique component of the SCI programme funded by the Gates Foundation: a tender process to encourage African pharmaceutical companies to formulate praziquantel so they could supply national control programmes, and the deliberate stimulation of an African market for praziquantel. (The topic was briefly touched on in Chapter 7.)

It may not have worked out quite how we hoped but, in a strange way, it succeeded – pharmaceutical companies did get involved and a reliable supply of praziquantel was made available to paralyse the worm.

The entire esoteric process of drug supply, from development through clinical trials, registration and drug pricing, could once have been said to be of little apparent interest to the general public, especially if you lived in a developed country. Access was assumed. This no longer holds – these matters have come to feature in news about COVID-19 vaccines or drug supplies from Europe to UK pharmacies post-Brexit, and the *British Medical Journal* can be found worrying about price hikes in drugs supplied to the UK's NHS (Morgan *et al.*, 2020). SCI's experience in this field should therefore be illuminating.

© Fenwick, Norris and McCall 2022. *A Tale of a Man, a Worm and a Snail: The Schistosomiasis Control Initiative* (A. Fenwick *et al.*)
DOI: 10.1079/9781786392558.0012

The SCI Plan – Better Access to Drugs

Clearly, the SCI programme was, and is, heavily dependent on widespread and easy access to praziquantel. With national programmes running in six countries (and a future with many more planned), we recognized the need for a global market with multiple producers of the drug bidding for African government tenders. This would be a major change from the situation in 2000 when there was virtually no African market. But manufacturers needed to see an adequate demand for praziquantel to make it worth their while to produce it, and there was a shortage of the funds in 2002 to encourage them. Endemic countries had no money to fund purchase, and there were no bilateral donors interested in NTDs – their focus was on malaria, HIV and TB.

So what could be an innovative model? SCI, supported by WHO, put forward a model to the Gates Foundation to create a competitive market for good-quality praziquantel, at reasonable prices, and establish a continuing supply to government-run disease-control programmes.

The Six-step Plan

We devised a six-point strategy which addressed the issues of competitive procurement, collaboration, information, registration, local formulation and donation (see Box 12.1).

Box 12.1. The six-step plan.

Procurement: Using guaranteed external financing (from the Gates Foundation) to procure praziquantel for six national schistosomiasis control programmes, SCI was able to interest several manufacturers and shape the market for praziquantel in Africa.

Collaboration: SCI used the availability of praziquantel to encourage collaboration with WHO and ministries of health to stimulate national demand for schistosomiasis control and for praziquantel.

Information: It was imperative that SCI improved available information about schistosomiasis and praziquantel – and publicize its safety, efficacy and low price.

Registration: Several manufacturers and drug companies were stimulated to provide the registration documents for praziquantel in endemic countries to create conditions for competitive tenders.

Local formulation: By purchasing the active ingredient and offering it to local pharmaceutical companies, SCI would try to stimulate the formulation of praziquantel in Africa by local manufacturers with good manufacturing practice (GMP) approval.

Donation: During 2003–2006, SCI would solicit donations of praziquantel from manufacturing companies and these additional drugs would be used to support additional coverage in the SCI country national control programmes.

Step 1: procurement and tenders

SCI was planning to purchase up to 50 million tablets to treat 20 million children.

Very little praziquantel was being purchased by countries but USAID had funded an 'NTD Project', which provided some more money for the purchase of the drug.

We were in a position, with the Gates funding, we hoped, to encourage multiple producers, which would lead to cheaper praziquantel; this, in turn, would build demand in other countries, thus encouraging even cheaper praziquantel. We reasoned that if they were Africa-based, prices and supply might be even more sustainable.

Sadly, the obvious candidate with experience, the Egyptian company EIPICO, did not seem interested to supply sub-Saharan Africa with praziquantel, which both surprised and disappointed me. In the end, it was only in Tanzania that local manufacture proved to be successful but this was for the internal market and not for other African countries, and it turned out to be a temporary situation for reasons that will become clear.

A particular hiccup occurred over tenders. Our hope was that procurement of local formulation (see later) might be handled by individual governments but we had to abandon this venture after an attempt to have one of the six countries run a tender. The price offers that came in from the suppliers were double what SCI was paying for praziquantel.

However, by 2008, there was a thriving market for praziquantel, with manufacturers from China, South Korea and India competing in the marketplace. Thus, in general terms, we can say that the plan was a success, albeit with a few hiccups on the way.

Step 2: collaboration

The second major strand of the SCI plan addressed partnering and partnerships. With a project as ambitious in scope as the SCI, little could be successfully achieved without the concerted effort of particular partnerships. By working with recognized global players dominant in the field of healthcare in developing countries, SCI and their partners raised awareness across different levels of society, from donor and recipient governments, and from foundations, to local endemic populations and the public. In raising awareness of our control programmes, we expected to build demand for them and thus for praziquantel, and so to encourage pharmaceutical companies to enter the praziquantel market. Three key players were the World Health Organization (WHO) and, in selected countries, the World Food Programme (WFP) and the World Bank.

WHO

The WHO has played a major role in setting global policy on schistosomiasis control for decades and has been a continuous central collaborator for SCI, achieved WHO GMP certification by January 2005. It was expected that these GMP-certified companies would explore opportunities to export their drugs to other markets in Africa.

In 2005, two of the Tanzanian pharmaceutical firms, Shelys and Tanzanian Pharmaceutical Industries Limited (TPI) did supply praziquantel to Tanzania at competitive prices, paid for by SCI. Despite Shelys building additional facilities in Dar es Salaam in 2006, they never managed to expand into exports and only ever supplied tablets for the local Tanzanian market.

As a result of our experience, we decided to abandon encouraging local formulation and local purchase and we continued to purchase from within the UK using donated funds. We then donated these drugs to recipient countries for their national programmes from 2003 to 2012, at which point a huge external donation from Merck Serono took over.

Step 6: donation

Huge donations changed the face of NTD control but scupper part of our plan!

In 2000, only three of the NTDs were covered by pharmaceutical donations.

Since 1986, Mectizan had been donated by Merck Sharp Dom in the USA through the Mectizan Donation Programme (MDP) in order to eliminate blindness due to onchocerciasis in Africa, and this donation was increased when it was shown that Mectizan in conjunction with albendazole could reduce the transmission of LF causative agents *Brugia malayi* and *Wucheraria bancrofti*.

GSK began their donation programme – albendazole against LF, in 1997 – and Pfizer launched a programme in 1999 against trachoma by donating Zithromax. All of these drugs needed to be delivered just once a year to many millions of infected and at-risk people in endemic areas using MDA.

In contrast to these three neglected diseases, schistosomiasis and STH had not been supported by any significant corporate donation programme prior to 2008. Bayer, the pharma company which originally developed praziquantel, resolutely and repeatedly refused to donate substantial quantities of the drug, although numerous approaches were made to them by WHO and others. Bayer's response was to donate only relatively small quantities of the drug to small-scale research projects in Africa, but they responded negatively to country requests for large numbers of praziquantel tablets and any long-term donation requests.

This was what had forced our hand; why we had hoped to build a competitive African market, and encourage local formulation and local purchase by national governments.

In 2004, SCI received donated praziquantel from an unexpected source. MedPharm stepped in and for three years donated praziquantel in quantities reaching a value of about $1 million per annum in 2004, 2005 and 2006. As has been explained (Chapter 7), this donation was curtailed by the change in the Canadian tax laws.

Then came the amazing Gates NTD day in January 2012 when Merck Serono (Merck KGaA) announced a massive increase in donated praziquantel.

Dream of a Competitive Market Fails

When SCI's dream of a long-term, competitive market for praziquantel, with several companies bidding to meet national government tenders, was not realized, we became dependent on donated praziquantel for treating children, and had to purchase praziquantel for any programmes where adults needed treatment.

Obviously, this changed in 2012 when Merck Serono stepped up to the plate, but at the time, the SCI team suffered a conflict between the realization of free drug donations on a massive scale and the nurturing of an open, local and competitive marketplace to supply Africa. We were very aware of the danger that the obvious merits of drug donations could be short-term as the donor may withdraw them.

However, because of the limited funding available for schistosomiasis control, there can be no doubting the advantageous benefit if the praziquantel donation remains long-term. Had the praziquantel donations remained at the 20 million tablets (to treat 8 million children) per year, which Merck originally donated, schistosomiasis prevalence would never have been controlled. WHO initially distributed these 20 million tablets to some (non-SCI supported) countries with the idea of encouraging new programmes to start up in countries that did not already have a schistosomiasis control project. Sadly, these countries lacked the infrastructure, resources and expertise to correctly distribute even the small number of tablets they received. The impact of the Merck donation would only become significant when the size and duration of the donation grew exponentially from the 20 million-tablet level. Once Merck Serono (also known as E. Merck) committed to the donation target of 250 million tablets annually, all the planned control programmes expanded.

Donated Praziquantel Encouraged Country Buy-in

The establishment of SCI programmes in the first six countries, using praziquantel purchased with the Gates award and supplemented by the MedPharm donation, supported 40 million treatments.

With hindsight, we can see that these results were significant enough to have stimulated interest from recipient countries and brought in other donors. Furthermore, though donation suppressed the market we were trying to open up, it was definitely a factor in growing the demand from African countries for national programmes.

Interestingly, whereas WHO had predicted a demand to cover all treatments (children and adults), what the countries actually wanted was treatment for their children, which has now been met by the Merck donation.

It was clear, in 2007, that donations of praziquantel by MedPharm would not continue, and indeed the Gates Foundation would cease to support the SCI schistosomiasis elimination programmes in Africa. So in retrospect we regard the Merck donation as a 'god-send'.

Since 2007, there has been a slow but sure positive change in the schistosomiasis treatment outreach and, at last, elimination targets for 2030 might just be met. It has to be said, that because of the scale needed, elimination is only going to be achievable through continued drug donation from global pharmaceutical companies.

13 Advocacy and Promotion of SCI Activity

Organ Damage Takes Years to Manifest

It can take many years from initial infection for the damage caused by schistosomiasis, particularly infection with *S. mansoni*, to be recognized. By the time symptoms are obvious, the consequences can be very serious and ultimately irreversible. When William, a 32-year-old fisherman from the shores of Lake Albert, died from schistosomiasis, his liver and spleen were so engorged with eggs and riddled with scar tissue that his body was too bloated to fit into a coffin. His mourning family had to wrap his body in a papyrus mat before lowering him into his grave.

Not all cases are so extreme, but if only a small percentage of the estimated 200 million people infected with schistosomiasis in Africa suffer this fate, then the toll is unacceptably high. Schistosomiasis eggs collect and damage organs slowly, day after day, without their function being impaired – until it's too late. Often it is only then that symptoms become apparent, and schistosomiasis is diagnosed.

Well-planned and Local Advocacy – The Key to Engagement

Although the political systems inherited by the East and West African countries in which SCI was working are significantly different, all remain culturally conservative and noticeably hierarchical. Hierarchies exist everywhere – maybe due to wealth, maybe based on politics, sometimes based on religion.

When we set out to use advocacy in Africa, at all levels we had to follow the same pyramid-like cascade of communication, as it filters through the hierarchy from ministry of health to local health professionals and ministry of education through teachers to children in school. The difference is that today it can happen much more quickly because of better FM radio coverage and mobile phones. We do also have to engage with and use local government because today, countries are divided into 'district health regions' (by whatever name) with populations from 50,000 up to half a million people in each.

© Fenwick, Norris and McCall 2022. *A Tale of a Man, a Worm and a Snail: The Schistosomiasis Control Initiative* (A. Fenwick *et al.*)
DOI: 10.1079/9781786392558.0013

For SCI, engaging senior officials within central government was the place to start, but we soon learned that this was just the beginning of a process. If we were to succeed in getting treatments to the rural population of a country, it was vital for someone, be it SCI teams or the in-country co-ordinators, to disseminate information at district level and reach out to key decision makers within local government.

Workshops – Education and Training

Advocacy workshops were essential, and at each we needed to introduce the topic of schistosomiasis (or bilharzia, if that's the name they knew) and worms. Incredibly, even in districts with a prevalence of more than 50% worm infestation in the population, the people were often hearing about these worms for the first time. Those that had heard of bilharzia and other worms were usually familiar with red urine or enlarged stomachs but would usually be ignorant of how the infection was transmitted. We would present an overview of the parasites' life cycles and the symptoms they caused, and speak of our ambition to make people better, targeting with our message the regional medical officers (RMO), regional directors of education (RDE), headmasters, health assistants, religious leaders and anyone who was in a position to be influential. Then we described how simple our implementation plan was, being based on distributing safe and effective pills just once a year.

Each education session was designed to give the local participants an opportunity to ask questions, and even input their ideas so we could tailor the grand plan to suit local requirements. Our plans, however, always adhered to the WHO guidelines for bilharzia treatment which, when we started, was to offer treatment to school-age children if the prevalence in a sample from the school was over 10% and under 50%. However, if the prevalence was over 50% in children, we offered treatment to the whole community, because this magic figure of 50% meant there was a serious bilharzia health problem in that area. Once the decision had been made to treat schools or communities, teachers were trained to dispense the drugs within their school, or each community was asked to select someone they trusted whom they felt had the sense of responsibility required and who was widely known to become a drug distributor. Whoever was selected was then offered individual training.

These open meetings were vital to achieve the required community compliance and participation and acceptance of the proposed drugs praziquantel and albendazole. They were designed to help villagers feel at ease with the distribution of pills, and give them an opportunity to ask questions. We could hear directly their concerns and try to dispel any mis-conceptions that may have had an adverse impact upon medicine uptake. People being offered free medication, especially those who are not sure that they are in fact ill, may question why they were being given drugs.

It was essential to deal with these issues before any misunderstandings started circulating widely amongst the community to the detriment of the programme.

We arranged for local radio stations to broadcast messages regarding treatment, written by the implementation team in collaboration with local authorities and, of course, in the appropriate language. That is not easy because in Uganda, FM radio stations are broadcasting in 70 different local languages! However, after all this publicity, drug compliance was reasonably successful.

Launch in Uganda – Making Use of Press Releases

The first national programme to tackle schistosomiasis (bilharzia) in sub-Saharan Africa was launched in Uganda by the Deputy Prime Minister, Brigadier Moses Ali. As you can see from the fulsome press release that follows, every detail was captured.

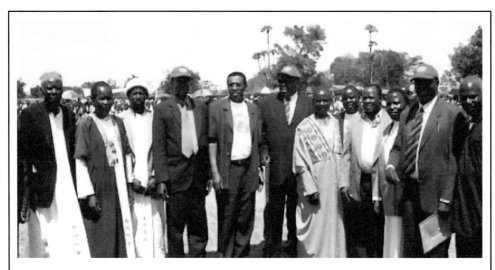

Fig. 13.1. The Deputy Prime Minister, the Honourable Brigadier Moses Ali with village elders.

The Ugandan Bilharzia and Worm Control Programme was officially launched on March 4th 2003 in Pakwach, Jonam County, Nebbi, a region particularly badly affected by schistosomiasis. The Deputy Prime Minister, Brigadier Moses Ali, represented the President, His Excellency Yoweri Kaguta Museveni. The ceremony was attended by several ministers plus officials from the Ugandan Central Government, and Eight Districts all endemic for schistosomiasis. From overseas there were guests from the Schistosomiasis Control Initiative (SCI) Imperial College London, the African Regional Office of the World Health Organisation, the Danish Bilharziasis Laboratory (DBL), and Save the Children.

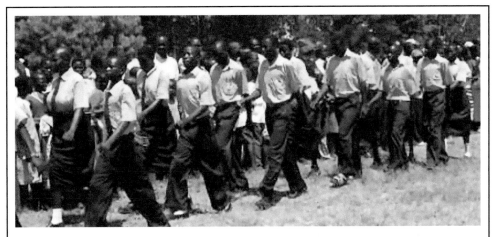

Fig. 13.2. The guests were greeted by a procession of schoolchildren.

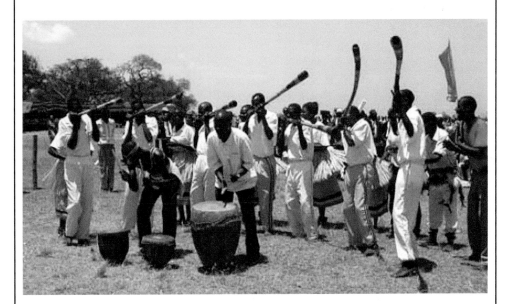

Fig. 13.3. There was music and dancing too!

A convoy of vehicles drove the 400 km from Kampala on the Monday, and on Tuesday morning, three aircraft flew in with 45 'VIP' guests. On arrival at Pakwach, ministers and guests were greeted by a lively procession of local school children and community members, accompanied by a musical fanfare from a trumpet and drum band. This was followed by dancing and entertainment, including an animated poem about schistosomiasis performed by local children. Exhibition stalls had been set up, providing educational material and information on schistosomiasis control and other health issues such as lymphatic filariasis, sexual health and Guinea Worm eradication. Guests were shown examples of health education materials, and looked down field microscopes to identify common parasites or eggs. They learned about transmission and control of common vector borne diseases and saw how the present initiative fits into a coherent scheme of health education and control programmes in Uganda.

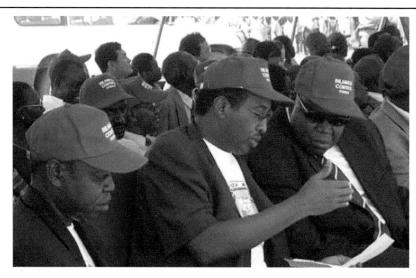

Fig. 13.4. (left to right) Hon. Fred Omach, MP for Nebbi, Brig. Jim Muhwezi, Minister of Health, and Deputy Prime Minister, Brigadier Moses Ali.

The guests then heard speeches from the Hon. Fred Omach, MP for Nebbi, the LCS (Director) of Nebbi District, Dr Narcis Kabatereine, the National Coordinator for the Bilharzia and Worm Control Program; Dr O. Walker the WHO WR for Uganda, Dr Alan Fenwick, Director of SCI, Dr Pascal Magnussen of DBL, and Hon. Brig. Jim Muhwezi, Minister of Health. The final speech was given by the Hon. Brig. Moses Ali the Deputy Prime Minister.

Professor Fenwick read a greeting from the Bill and Melinda Gates Foundation, and then described schistosomiasis in Uganda as "a supreme example of a disease suffered by the poorest of the poor" and commented that "in creating a successful prevention and treatment programme that can be emulated in countries round the world, the Schistosomiasis Control Initiative has an opportunity to make a major impact in the fight against schistosomiasis worldwide." He stated his hope that the success of this programme will improve nutrition and health in children, prolong life-expectancy among those affected and prevent unnecessary suffering and disability.

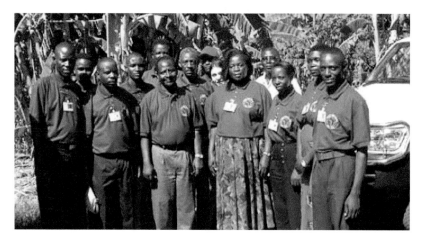

Fig. 13.5. The Ugandan field team.

Dr Kabatereine described the impact of schistosomiasis in Uganda and reviewed the progress that has been made in tackling the disease to date. He thanked the donors, the Bill and Melinda Gates Foundation, and welcomed the availability of affordable drugs, which has enabled a mass treatment programme to be realised. He then described the Bilharzia and Worm Control Programme, which will involve 4–5 years of mass treatment using donated drug supplies, followed by a sustained effort by the Ugandan government to take over and continue the control programme. The national programme will be implemented by the Ugandan Ministry of Health in collaboration with the Vector Control Division, the SCI at Imperial College, London and other NGOs.

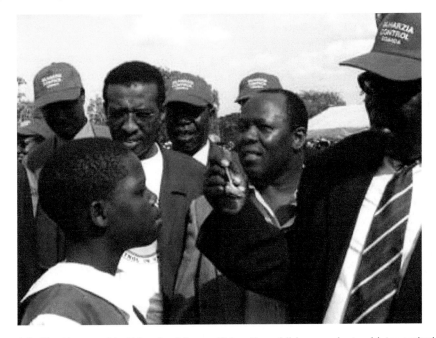

Fig. 13.6. The Honourable Brigadier Moses Ali treating children against schistosomiasis and STH.

In an appropriate finale to the official launch, several children were treated against schistosomiasis and STH (using praziquantel and albendazole respectively) by the Brig. Moses Ali, to demonstrate how easy treatment can be.

Brig Moses then handed over cartons of drugs to the Director of Health Services of eight districts; Arua, Adjumani, Gulu, Hoima, Moyo, Masindi, Nebbi and Wakiso. Each of these districts received sufficient drug to treat 30,000 people. Drugs will soon be collected from the National Medical Stores by ten more districts. It is envisaged that within a year at least one million infected and at-risk individuals in Uganda will receive treatment.

Finally, I spoke to emphasize that this programme belonged to the Ugandan people, and expressed hope that the level of support shown at the launch, from the politicians, NGOs, local and religious leaders, teachers and community members would help the programme get off to a flying start and contribute to its success.

Promoting SCI's Work in Uganda on Film (Andy Jillings)

The Ugandan launch had been such a success that I accepted an opportunity to have a short promotion film made; and again, luck played its part. Shortly after joining Imperial College, the Department of Infectious Disease Epidemiology organized a two-day weekend meeting in the Lake District which Margie and I decided to join to get to know some of the department people we had not yet met.

The people we bonded with on the walks around the Lakes were Dr Maria Gloria Basanez, who worked on onchocerciasis transmission modelling, and her husband Andy Jillings, who turned out to be an independent documentary maker.

While walking around the beautiful countryside we developed a plan for Andy to make a documentary film highlighting the work that SCI was doing in Uganda and was hoping to do in the future. Andy was an amazing man and his attention to detail was, I soon realized, an essential characteristic to the success of making a film. We had a thrilling visit to Uganda where Andy met Dr Narcis Kabatereine (of course) but also the then Minister of Finance, the Honourable Fred Jachan-Omach Mandir, who became a really good friend and supporter of SCI's work in Uganda. Fred came from, and was the MP for, Pakwach, which was in West Nile, a heavily infected area of Uganda. Andy also found an individual who was suffering from acute schistosomiasis. He came over very movingly on camera when telling his story of how schistosomiasis had affected him and his family because he was too ill to fish and therefore he was unable to earn a living to feed the family. Andy filmed some fabulous footage of people fishing, of the treatment campaign and health education sessions. His documentary was 20 minutes long but he kindly also made a shorter three-minute summary film and both were widely distributed on CD in the early days of SCI and used for publicity and advocacy purposes.

I do not see too much of Andy these days but I will never forget him and thank him for his dedication and support for SCI over the years.

Public Engagement Strategy in Niger

In Niger, we only needed to prepare advocacy in one language – French. Our messages went out with several social mobilization national radio announcements and television advertisements, publicizing the mass treatment campaign. At the regional and district level, community radio stations were used to disseminate the social mobilization messages developed by the PNLBG (the national programme against bilharzia) to ensure extensive coverage of the target population. In addition, the PNLBG also worked directly with regional and district (health and education) officials to further disseminate the messages about target groups, transmission and the mass treatment campaign to local target populations. Village chiefs, village criers,

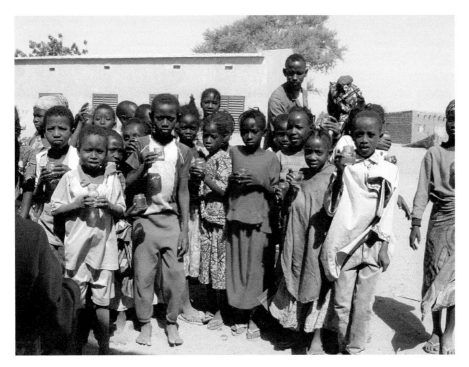

Fig. 13.7. Niger children with their urine samples.

community drug distributors and teachers were also asked to circulate the messages about the drug distribution prior to the mass treatment campaign.

We could not be faulted for trying to use every means possible to get the message across.

The launching of these programmes was designed to maximize publicity but also to allay any fears about the drugs causing harm. The public declaration that the medicines were free was designed to prevent people being

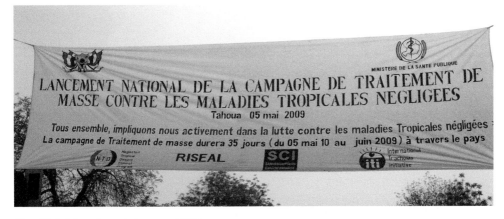

Fig. 13.8. Niger launch banner 2009.

charged money by any unscrupulous officers, and indeed, we felt we had inspired confidence in the programmes.

Offering and Implementing SCI In-country Assistance – Summary

I made it a rule to only approach a country's ministry of health once I could guarantee available funding and drugs for that country for at least two years. Once this had been confirmed, I would visit the country to offer access to the medicines plus financial and technical assistance. I would ask the assistance of our WHO colleagues to make an approach to senior ministry of health staff. SCI would then offer to participate at the start of the programme by mapping the distribution of both diseases (schistosomiasis and STH), and in partnership, to assist the government to prepare and implement an agreed treatment plan with a target to scale up to national programme level. That's it in a nutshell!

We arrive prepared to provide essential equipment for mapping, such as microscopes and laboratory supplies for stool and urine examination, and offer training of laboratory technicians in how to collect samples and

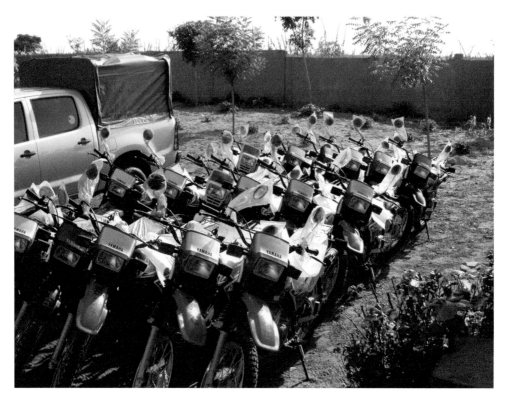

Fig. 13.9. Niger motorbikes donation.

examine them. For implementation, we would provide items such as dose poles, motorbikes, vehicles, fuel, etc. if needed. For baseline data collection, we would provide height poles, weighing machines, lancets for taking blood samples, and haemocue machines to measure haemaglobin to detect anaemia. Many of these items are funded jointly by the ministries and the SCI, but once purchased, they belong completely to that country. Other costs that we might meet are staff members' daily field allowances for the training and treatment days, and a daily allowance during implementation of the public health programme. By working in partnership with local ministry of health employees, the gradual handover of programme management to the country itself is intended to be as smooth as possible.

Developing In-country Capacity

In each country where we worked, the SCI, as do other NTD programmes, placed emphasis on strengthening healthcare services within countries so that governments could effectively pick up treatment programmes once the external support for preliminary treatment rounds had been completed.

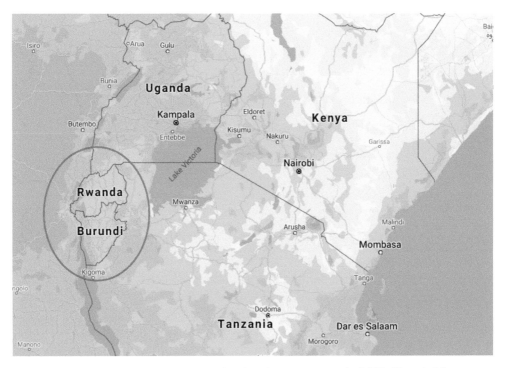

Fig. 13.10. Rwanda and Burundi were added to the programme in 2007. (Google Maps, created 2021.)

The SCI had a total of just 20 staff, consisting of a core managerial group and a financial team, supporting programme managers allocated to work with countries. The more resources we attracted, the more expansion to more countries was possible, and this led to hiring of more programme managers. From 2003 to 2007, six countries benefitted from our support. We added Burundi and Rwanda in 2007 (Fig. 13.10).

By 2015, SCI was contributing to the NTD programmes in 16 countries. Each of our home-based programme managers was allocated to overseeing activity in at least two countries. Other than the UK-based programme managers, the SCI focuses on developing capacity sourced from within a country's ministries of health and education. Local staff members from the central ministries and districts become partners, and health workers and teachers from the villages themselves are trained participants in the control and elimination programmes with responsibility for delivering the treatment to the villagers.

14 M&E – What Is Measured, and Reaching Out to Donors

Well-planned M&E allows us to not only justify investment but also helps to provide quantifiable evidence for future donors. It enables researchers to track progress against disease in terms of prevalence, and intensity and levels of morbidity. Measuring and documenting real and in-kind costs is an essential part of M&E, since other development needs to compete with treatment for limited resources. For example, drilling and installing a well can cost between $4,000 and $12,000. Our argument to support MDA is that other health interventions cannot compare in terms of cost-effectiveness with the cost of an NTD treatment of between 10 and 50 cents per person per annum.

So what do we measure? We measure egg count, morbidity (damage to organs, anaemia, stunting) and impact on cognition.

Egg Count and Probable Pathology

Variability of the consequences of infection

The mortality, morbidity and pathology due to schistosomiasis varies from person to person because each person is harbouring a different number of worms, which in turn means that inside each person a different number of eggs are laid daily. The number of worms is determined by the frequency and duration of exposure to infection and/or to genetic factors, and we assume that the more worms there are, the more eggs are laid and the quicker the serious consequences of infection are noticed.

The best, and indeed the only, indicator of the number of worms in any one individual is measured by the 'intensity of infection'; that is the number of eggs found in the urine or stool. The rule of thumb is that the only early symptoms which will be detected are blood in the urine caused by *S. haematobium*. Early symptoms from *S. mansoni* are, potentially, blood in the stool, but this is harder to detect. In most infected people, the many and varied serious consequences caused by both species of schistosomiasis can take years to become detectable.

© Fenwick, Norris and McCall 2022. *A Tale of a Man, a Worm and a Snail: The Schistosomiasis Control Initiative* (A. Fenwick *et al.*)
DOI: 10.1079/9781786392558.0014

Mitigation of infection in children – praziquantel must target children

Because most infections seem to be contracted during childhood and symptoms can take 10–15 years after initial exposure to manifest, it is vital for us to be proactive and reach out to children during their school-age years, to offer treatment as early as possible after they are infected, which is before any discernible symptoms have appeared.

Praziquantel is a wonder drug but we need to remember that it does not kill the immature worms, it only kills the adults. But killing the adult worms stops the laying of eggs, which immediately stops the progression of organ damage. Apart from blood in the urine (*S. haematobium*), the early stages of infections may be unnoticed, so health education messages are needed so that parents and children understand what the infection is doing to them, despite no apparent symptoms, and will accept the treatment we offer.

Morbidity – Measuring the Effect on the Individual

Morbidity due to schistosomiasis is an altogether more complicated aspect of disease impact and therefore difficult to measure accurately. There are many different possible effects of the worms and their eggs on the human body, and it is difficult to select which clinical features to measure in the rural environment where most schistosomiasis and STH-related disease occurs. Ideally, morbidity measurements would provide an indication of how the disease affects the body's organs and would provide a quantitative and reproducible measure of morbidity.

All we can do is look for certain symptoms and decide whether they have been due to schistosomiasis or something else. Examples of what we might look for are lack of growth (height and weight), blood in the urine or stool, tender or enlarged liver and spleen, diarrhoea and anaemia. Very late stages of infection would lead to liver fibrosis, ascites, fibrosis of the bladder, bladder cancer and oesophageal varices and vomiting of blood.

Anaemia

Data indicates that in the developing world, 42% of children under five and 53% aged 5–14 are anaemic. The condition, which is very debilitating, reduces future work capacity, impairs ability to conduct daily activities, produces poor pregnancy outcomes and reduces cognitive functioning.

While anaemia and the consequences of anaemia may all be caused by schistosomiasis, they cannot be attributed solely to schistosomiasis. Malnutrition due to poverty and malaria are other common causes of anaemia. Equally, stunting can be caused by STH infections and schistosomiasis but stunting may be confounded by other conditions such as diet and co-parasitic infections. Anaemia can be measured and assessed by using a haemoglobinometer (Haemacue) to measure levels of haemoglobin, the protein in red blood cells which transports oxygen around the body.

Given the possible contribution by other infectious diseases (so-called 'confounding factors'), it is still considered that anaemia is a proven and reliable indicator of morbidity in a school-age child population. This is supported by evidence which suggests that peak prevalence and intensity of schistosomiasis occurs in 10- to 15-year olds which also coincides with a period of high iron demand for growth (Stephenson, 1993). Schistosomiasis is believed to deprive the body of this vital mineral.

Liver, bladder and spleen

Measuring liver enlargement and fibrosis, and looking for bladder fibrosis, are not only important for the individual patient, but also because they give us a true measure of schistosomiasis pathology among the population. Prior to the emergence of new technology, enlargement of liver and spleen were detected by palpation, but this is certainly not accurate and is open to observer error, which makes it risky to use the results definitively. The development and availability of portable ultrasound machines has made examinations more sensitive and accurate (Vennervald and Dunne, 2004).

Ultrasonography is therefore currently the diagnostic tool of choice for detecting disease-related conditions such as dilatation of the renal pelvis, bladder wall lesions, liver enlargement and fibrosis, and dilatation of the portal vein which runs between the intestine and the liver. The advantage of ultrasonography is its versatility under field conditions as well as the hospital setting. It provides a non-invasive procedure that is relatively simple for experienced technicians to perform, is well-accepted by communities, and provides a direct and quantitative image of pathologic changes. It provides sensitive and precise measurements of both *S. mansoni*- and *S. haematobium*-associated pathologic changes.

Height and weight

Other parameters which are obvious to measure are height and weight since heavy schistosomiasis and STH infections can cause malnutrition and stunting. However, we must remember that both anaemia *per se* and infection with worms are conditions typical of poverty, and the stunting could be due to malnutrition caused by poverty.

Impact on cognition and school attendance

Ideally, the SCI monitoring and evaluation would have tried to assess how the programme affected cognitive function and school attendance as well as the socio-economic achievements of those treated. However, to date, these parameters have not been examined by our M&E team due to logistical difficulties. Instead, we look to studies done by other research groups elsewhere. These provide strong evidence of the detrimental effects of STH infection on cognition and school attendance. Of these, hookworms (*Necator* and *Ancylostoma* species), whipworm (*Trichuris*) and roundworm (*Ascaris*) are the most common and important STHs in humans.

In addition to weakness and inability to physically walk the distance to school, infection with STH is documented to affect the neuropsychiatric activities of children. This condition damages school performance, although the mechanisms by which this happens are unclear. There are clinical studies that suggest that STH adversely affect cognition and memory and may even lower intelligence (Hotez, 2008; Nokes *et al.*, 1992; Sakti *et al.*, 1999).

Data from long-term studies demonstrates that the earning power of children who have grown up with heavy STH infections has been compromised (Ahuja *et al.*, 2017).

SCI Collected Data and Findings

In a programme as extensive as that conducted by the SCI, M&E activity needs to be conducted on a wide scale across each of the participant countries.

M&E: anaemia and schistosomiasis in Burkina Faso

SCI has investigated anaemia and its association with uro-genital schistosomiasis. In a study of 1727 children from 16 schools in Burkina Faso the relationship between *S. haematobium* infection and associated morbidity in children before and after treatment with praziquantel and albendazole (against STH) gave up some powerful results. Children with higher *S. haematobium* infection intensities proved to be more likely to present with severe haematuria (traces of blood, or gross blood, in urine), which suggests a correlation between heavy intensities of *S. haematobium* infection and anaemia and haematuria. The same study also provided evidence that heavy infections of uro-genital schistosomiasis are associated with lower haemaglobin concentrations and, therefore, with potential anemia.

When the children were followed a year later, after one round of treatment with praziquantel, they showed a significant reduction in the prevalence and intensity of infection of *S. haematobium* as well as a drop in the percentage of children with haematuria (Koukounari *et al.*, 2007).

M&E: sampling in Niger

In Niger, baseline data was collected from 1701 children and 483 adults in eight villages over the course of 2005 and 2006. The method of selection of villages and schools for monitoring was key to obtaining an accurate understanding of a programme's impact. The eight villages were in eight different districts in four

Demonstrating Value for Money and Economic Impact

As with most healthcare interventions, the strength of the health-economic argument can make or break a project and, if cost-effective, the programme will prove to be sustainable. The bottom line for treatment programmes is usually how much it costs relative to the benefit gained. It is also helpful for all decision makers, including national disease control co-ordinators, health planners and government policy-makers to have a cost breakdown of the programme to ensure that feasible and sustainable budgets are developed. For sustainable development, governments of SCI-supported countries require all the relevant costs that a ministry of health would need to assume if they were planning their own treatment campaign. Assessing the health-economic argument for a treatment campaign is complex, but is of growing importance in guiding health policy, planning and priority setting. Equally, from SCI's point of view, the data showing the cost-effectiveness of the control led to investment in SCI by foundations and individuals.

Uganda: SCI cost-effectiveness 2003–2010

Data on cost-effectiveness of schistosomiasis and STH treatment in Africa had been very limited prior to the establishment of SCI. We were able to collate, evaluate and publish data for the years 2003–2010.

A study we conducted in Uganda assessed cost per child and cost per case of anaemia averted, providing some indication of the cost benefit related to helminth control treatment. Data was collected through interviews with district officials and from accounting records in six of the 23 treatment districts. Both financial and economic costs were assessed and estimated to provide, in US dollars, the cost per schoolchild treated and cost per case of anaemia averted. The results showed that the overall economic cost per child treated in the six districts was US$0.54 and the cost-effectiveness was US$3.19 per case of anaemia averted.

As expected, the researchers found that the price varied with the number of children treated, indicating the effect of economy of scale. They also found that cost-effectiveness varied with the district (Brooker *et al.*, 2008).

Harnessing Political Will and Capturing Media Attention

At the time that the Gates Foundation funding was coming to an end for SCI's work we were able to secure one last tranche of funding for global awareness of NTDs. We (Imperial College) were therefore delighted to be approached by a television company to make a contribution to a new documentary series, *Survival*, on diseases of the developing world.

Survival – TV and the global health debate

The television production company, Rockhopper TV, had secured funding from the Gates Foundation to produce an eight-programme series to be aired on BBC World, weekly, during 2010. Each programme addressed an issue related to improving health and well-being for people in the world's poorest countries. The issues looked at were schistosomiasis, hookworm, sleeping sickness, malaria, air pollution, maternal health, child health, TB and HIV, and the programmes were concluded with a one-hour televised public debate.

As an introduction to the series, the BBC invited me to be interviewed by Stephen Sackur in a programme called *Hard Talk*, also shown weekly on BBC World. I expected this to be a friendly discussion, with Stephen giving me some idea of the questions in advance. This did not happen, and I was given no warning of the questions so I had to think quickly and be very careful to be accurate with my responses.

Tremendous credit is due to Richard Wilson and Anya Sitaram (his wife), the owners of Rockhopper TV, for the series. Over a period of ten weeks, thanks to them, the world audience of BBC World were given a wide introduction to neglected tropical diseases. I heard from a number of people who had seen my *Hard Talk* interview, but none more surprising than our friends from Chalfont St Giles who were on holiday in Zanzibar. He said he had switched on the BBC to get the football scores, only to see me!

I have been lucky to own a dog

One aspect of the TV series *Survival* which had slipped by me during the planning of the TV programmes was a Gates Foundation request that the impact of the programmes be determined by some mechanism of evaluation. When the project manager at Gates asked about our plan, I admitted that I had not, in fact, developed one, and actually did not quite understand what they wanted from us, or who could do it. The Foundation flew myself and Richard Wilson (Richard W.) to Washington, DC, where we met with Kathy, our contact there, and she laid out some possibilities for evaluation both in the UK, Europe and internationally. As for who might put this together, she suggested Ipsos-Mori, the organization I knew as the one that predicts who will win our general election.

Kathy came up with a plan to help us because it turned out that Richard Silman, the European Manager of Ipsos-Mori, was in Seattle for a few days negotiating a contract with the Foundation, and she thought that, if successful, he would throw in the evaluation we needed for a small extra surcharge. Kathy set off back to Seattle and said she would e-mail the result of her meeting with Richard Silman. Richard W. and I headed back to the UK, happy that things would work out for us to evaluate the programmes.

As she promised, on the following Monday morning, Kathy e-mailed that Richard Silman was happy to sign with me to evaluate the programmes and we should meet to plan the details. I immediately e-mailed him and asked when we could meet and he suggested the next morning.

Unfortunately, I had a golf knock-out game fixed for 8 am and so I asked if we could meet in the afternoon, but Richard replied that he could not because he was flying to Stuttgart at 1 pm for a few days. It was a bit embarrassing because I did not really want to show that a game of golf was more important than a Gates contract, but at that moment it was! He agreed that we could meet the following week when he was back in London. So in order to play golf at 8 am I had to go out extra early with the dog (Simba, our yellow Labrador) and walk him at 6 am in the fields near our house. I was not expecting to see my usual dog-walking friends so early, but there was a man and his dog on a lead, someone I had never met before. As we passed each other I suggested we let the dogs run free and have a romp, which we agreed to do, and off they went. I said I had not seen him or his dog before and he said he did not usually use this field to walk in, nor so early.

'Trouble is,' he said, 'I have to fly to Stuttgart this afternoon.'

'Is your name Richard by any chance,' I asked? He looked at me in amazement and both of us have dined out many times on that incredible coincidence ever since.

He was indeed the European Director for Ipsos-Mori and he had flown in from Seattle just two days previously having agreed to do our evaluation. He lives just two streets from one side of the field and I lived two streets on the other side. Ipsos-Mori went on to evaluate the impact of the programmes for us in the UK, Germany and Japan.

Years 2007–2012: SCI Loses Some But Wins Much More

Having established the schistosomiasis programmes in Burkina Faso and Niger in 2003, and then sub-contracted with RTI to continue their support using USAID funding, SCI then lost USAID support for Burkina Faso and Mali. This happened because during the second USAID funding phase, ITI's support to Mali and SCI's to Burkina Faso and Niger was transferred from RTI to FHI. FHI then decided to rebid the support to these countries, and instead of continuing with SCI, despite our long and successful history of parasite control in these countries, they awarded their sub-contract to Helen Keller International. This was probably because HKI was US-based while SCI was UK-based.

SCI reaches out to new donors and moves into 13 new countries

Despite this disappointing setback, SCI did thrive by reaching out to new donors and moving to work in new countries. The data we had gathered from our M&E of the existing programmes proved invaluable in helping us

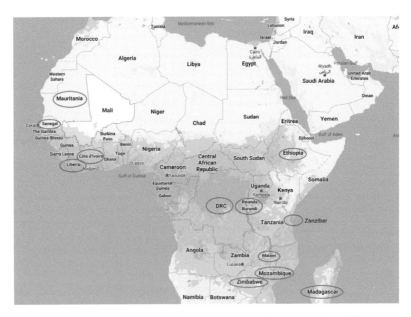

Fig. 14.2. Established SCI programmes in Africa. (Google Maps, created 2021)

to reach out and make a solid case to new donors including several high-net-worth individuals, which, when added to the new money from the British government (DFID), helped us to establish schistosomiasis control programmes in Burundi, Cote D'Ivoire, DRC, Ethiopia, Liberia, Madagascar, Malawi, Mauritania, Mozambique, Rwanda, Senegal, Zanzibar and Zimbabwe (Fig. 14.2).

The Target for Schistosomiasis: Not Eradication but Elimination or Control

Unfortunately, the word eradication is often wrongly used because eradication, in the public health context, means a permanent removal of the disease from the planet. We are targeting control in the first instance followed by elimination, which means an area has achieved local elimination.

Sadly, several species of animals have been eradicated but only one disease has been eradicated so far, and that is smallpox, thanks to vaccination. Polio was a scourge, globally, in the mid-20th century but with the vaccine developed by Sabin, eradication became a target.

Funding from the Gates Foundation and the Rotary movement, among others, encouraged the WHO to declare the first target of 1995 to rid the planet of polio. As it stands now, in 2020/21, polio is not quite eradicated but there are very few new cases, and only Pakistan and Afghanistan remain countries with wild polio cases. Africa, in August 2020, was declared free of wild polio, which, even if 25 years late, is a tremendous achievement.

Epidemiologists and mathematical modellers all agree that it is unlikely that schistosomiasis and STH will be eradicated for a very long time, and certainly not until there is a socio-economic upturn with better sanitation and clean water supplies introduced into all endemic areas. However, local elimination is certainly possible and is the current target in many countries (WHO has published plans for programme managers), accepting that some hot spots of infection will probably remain with these needing further regular treatment. Already in some areas, MDA has dramatically reduced prevalence as measured by structured monitoring and evaluation.

15 Building Partnerships – High Stakes for High Rewards

Time to Make Progress

Poverty, disease and donors

A reminder of the situation in the year 2000: one-sixth of the world's population were suffering from one or more NTDs. Given that most of these diseases are both preventable and treatable, they could and should be eliminated. That they were still so widespread equates to one billion people needlessly suffering debilitation, disfigurment and long-term harmful consequences to health and socio-economic stability. Unfortunately, these were also the neediest group of people on our planet, receiving the least attention in terms of economic development, which meant that they suffered from a lack of clean water supplies, adequate sanitation, schools and health facilities, and financial support from the wealthier members of the public or from local governments.

As mentioned earlier, these rural populations remained largely ignored because they lived in locations far from urban centres and were therefore difficult to reach. Some say that they are not looked after better because politicians do not benefit from their votes. Indeed, the clear majority of the world's more affluent people are ignorant of, and therefore uncaring about, their plight. The stratum of society affected by these diseases is so poor that they are often isolated from the rest of society and not considered for investment or redemption. In fact, the link between poverty and the prevalence of NTDs is so strong that it has been used as a proxy indicator of socio-economic status (WHO speech of Director General Margaret Chan, March 2007). Relative to the very public and media-friendly attention given to the plight of people suffering from the 'big three' diseases, the NTDs receive very few column inches, and, prior to 2002, very little financial help.

The few NTD leaders worked together to bring donor countries, pharmaceutical companies and other donors on board to build on the progress made using the initial Gates Foundation funding.

Thanks to our advocacy and the early results of our work, people learned what these diseases were, how many were infected and affected, and realized how harmful these diseases can be to every country's economy.

© Fenwick, Norris and McCall 2022. *A Tale of a Man, a Worm and a Snail: The Schistosomiasis Control Initiative* (A. Fenwick *et al.*)
DOI: 10.1079/9781786392558.0015

The NTD message was refined so that the people with influence, whom we needed to alert, were shown images of seriously affected individuals *and* educated on how inexpensive annual NTD treatments can be. The horrific photographs shocked at least some of them into action, and a lot of credit for this improved advocacy goes to the Global Network for Neglected Tropical Diseases Control (GNNTDC).

Box 15.1. NTD control programmes within the GNNTDC.

International Trachoma Initiative: Founded in 1998, the ITI quickly reached 10 million in 11 countries but has since expanded after the mapping initiative to reach 160 million people annually. The ITI approach consists of targeted support of country programmes for expanded implementation of the SAFE strategy – Surgery, Antibiotics (Zithromax donated by Pfizer), Face-washing, and Environmental change – to eliminate disease. Some countries are close to completing their annual programmes and trachoma is close to elimination in several countries.

Schistosomiasis Control Initiative: The SCI delivered 40 million treatments for schistosomiasis and STH in 2007 with Gates Foundation funding but planned further expansion into 16 countries with support from DFID, Legatum, Giving What We Can, GiveWell and many private, small and high-net-worth individual donors. SCI continued to support countries to treat over 40 million individuals per annum and by 2019 had passed the milestone of over 200 million treatments against schistosomiasis.

Global Alliance to Eliminate Lymphatic Filariasis: GAELF was launched in 1999 and had a target to reach over 100 million people with lymphatic filariasis (also known as elephantiasis) in Africa. The organization reached 45 million in 2006/7, but suffered temporary constraints in 2007 related to distribution cost resources. Merck and GlaxoSmithKline donate Mectizan and albendazole to the programme. By 2019, almost all 70 endemic countries had started control programmes and several countries in Africa had reached the end of seven years' treatments and were ready to stop annual MDA.

African Programme for Onchocerciasis Control: Formed in 1996, APOC had been reaching 40 million every year. Its target is 80 million in 19 countries. River blindness (onchocerciasis) was initially tackled in the 1970s by control of the vector blackfly with, initially, DDT and later more 'acceptable' insecticides (OCP). After 1985, treatment used donated Mectizan (courtesy of Merck). For 20 years, river blindness control has been an outstanding success but expansion of treatment was still required. With the demise of APOC in 2015 a new organization, ESPEN, was founded to carry forward the expansion of integrated treatment of NTDs in Africa.

Helen Keller International: Founded in 1915, HKI's mission was to save the sight of the most vulnerable. This mission therefore includes working to control and eliminate trachoma and onchocerciasis.

Task Force for Child Survival and Development: Founded in 1984 by Dr Foege, the Task Force today is based in Decator, Georgia, and includes NTD programmes such as Children without Worms, ITI, the Mectizan Donation Program and the NTD Support Center.

The Earth Institute at Columbia University: When we were discussing launching the GNNTDC, Peter Hotez asked Professor Jeffrey Sachs and his wife Sonia to join, and they hosted the first meeting of the group. They were not implementers but participated as policy advisors, and have supported the advocacy against NTDs ever since.

Founding of the Global Network for NTD Control, 2006

While we were working to implement the USAID programme, our group of parasitologists discussed getting together in a formal partnership to raise the profile of neglected diseases and to stimulate a paradigm shift in neglected disease control efforts. The rationale for integrating programmes seemed to make sense and the potential benefits were clear, so after a series of meetings between different NTD organizations and experts in the field, the GNNTDC was launched in September 2006.

The GNNTDC consisted of eight well-established organizations and was based at the Sabin Vaccine Institute in Washington, DC. The founding members were the George Washington University, the Earth Institute at Columbia University, the Liverpool School of Tropical Medicine, Helen Keller International, the International Trachoma Initiative, the Schistosomiasis Control Initiative, and the Task Force for Child Survival and Development. Collectively, we initiated a plan to implement integrated drug administration programmes across sub-Saharan Africa. Box 15.1 describes the NTD organizations participating in the GNNTDC.

GNNTDC Advocacy for the Cause of NTD Integrated Control

The first task for the GNNTDC was to develop stronger advocacy to bring the NTDs to the attention of the general public in developed countries and to

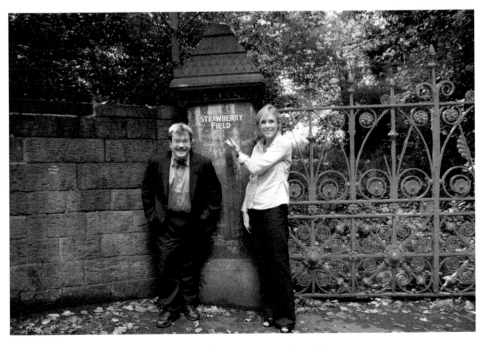

Fig. 15.1. Strawberry Field, Liverpool – Peter Hotez and Kari Stoever.

decision makers globally. What could we do for the NTDs? Professors Peter Hotez, David Molyneux and I brought them to the attention of Professor Jeffrey Sachs who had worked so hard with the Secretary General of the UN, Kofi Anan, to publicize the Millennium Development Goals (MDGs). The founding members of the GNNTDC held our first meeting with Jeffrey Sachs at Columbia University.

Initial funding for the GNNTDC was provided by Sabin and then by the Gates Foundation. The first grant – the first of many, we hoped – came from Geneva Global with funds from Legatum. Legatum had decided to fund NTD control in Burundi and Rwanda through SCI, and agreed to use GNNTDC as the secretariat for the grant because of the network being sited in the USA and relatively close to Geneva Global.

Much of the credit for the early success of the GNNTDC was due to the advocacy in Washington by Professor Peter Hotez and Ms Kari Stoever, who contacted several senators and representatives in the US government and also ensured attendance at high-profile events such as meetings of the Clinton Global Initiative. GNNTDC staff were successful in further raising the profile of NTDs, and funding for control, with advertising films and cartoons.

The GNNTDC was wound up in 2015 having served its purpose.

Donors Join Our Fight Against NTDs (2006–2012)

I am pleased to say that with the end of the Gates Foundation support in sight, at least to SCI for schistosomiasis, several other donors recognized the value of joining the fight against these diseases. The first donors to seriously support the NTD control programmes were the American government (USAID) and the British government (DFID).

The requests that we made to the bilateral donors in the developed world were for a long-term commitment to provide medicines, funding for mapping, annual treatment campaigns, and for post-treatment monitoring and reporting of the effects of the treatment back to the donors – basically, to expand what the Gates Foundation had started. The sad fact is that only USAID and DFID responded positively because the others did not want to be tied in to the large-scale, indefinite commitment that continued treatment demands.

To emphasize the extent of support received by all of us involved in NTD implementation, USAID, which in 2006 allocated $100 million over five years to tackle NTDs across eight sub-Saharan countries, later added more support, namely an increase in the allocation to $450 million globally. They gave a further $175 million in 2018, using RTI as the prime contractor. Their support, in general, went to different countries from the DFID funds.

DFID followed the USAID lead and allocated £50 million in 2008, increasing the commitment to £245 million in 2012, and then a further £200 million in 2019. These funds were shared between SCI, the Liverpool School of Tropical Medicine and, latterly, Sightsavers.

In engaging with 'prospective' donors, we soon learned that it is necessary, indeed imperative, to be open, honest and careful with our predictions and promises of what we can achieve. It is important that our achievement targets for each of the NTDs are focused to ensure that donor participation and plans to leverage longer-term funding from governments are factored into their giving from the beginning.

We (SCI in particular), but the other GNNTDC members also, strived to make our supported programmes sustainable by promoting local ownership and attempting to ensure the local staff resources, which would be needed for the long term, would be supported by locally allocated finance after the outside help has run its course.

Life After Gates – SCI Finds New Funding Partners

By the time the end of the Gates funding was in sight, SCI had achieved our initial goals and had a successful project with excellent results to publicize, as did our NTD colleagues working in parallel on lymphatic filariasis, onchocerciasis and trachoma. Indeed, the work of SCI by 2006 had been recognized in Burkina Faso and Niger with the award of medals to senior SCI staff, and I had been honoured by the Royal Society of Tropical Medicine and Hygiene with the award of the McKay Medal, a recognition of all that SCI staff had achieved.

After the funding from USAID and DFID for all the NTDs (more about this later), SCI developed separate partnerships and donations just for schistosomiasis and STH from private funders and charities, some from

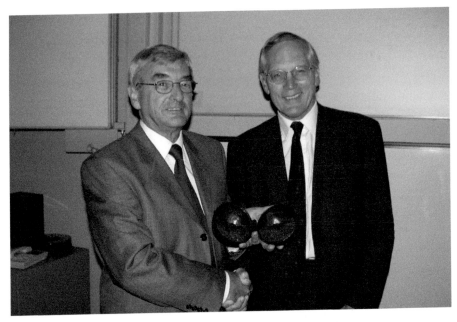

Fig. 15.2. The McKay Medal being received by Alan on behalf of SCI.

unexpected sources. A charity called Legatum, in 2006, provided funds to GNNTDC and SCI for schistosomiasis in Burundi and Rwanda. How this happened is a worthy tale in itself, but let me introduce it by way of mentioning two significant organizations in the story of SCI.

GiveWell and Giving What We Can

SCI owes much to two organizations, GiveWell and Giving What We Can, which evaluate charities for their members and advise them on which, in their opinion, promote better health and alleviate poverty. After a detailed examination of SCI's work and accounts in 2010, both named SCI as one of their top recommendations as a worthy recipient of their members' donations. This resulted in an increasing number of private wealthy individuals ('high-net-worth') and private foundations supporting SCI through small monthly donations or larger annual donations. Every year since, SCI has been subjected to detailed examination of their finances and achievements, and has remained a top recommendation for over ten consecutive years. Key supporters who came to us via these organizations include Thomas Mather (MaxMind) and Luke Ding (see Acknowledgements and Chapter 21) for more about them, particularly Luke.

But the major tale, a bit of a shaggy-dog story, is how we acquired Legatum, our first philanthropist after Bill Gates, and how this changed the NTD story.

Legatum – First Major Philanthropist to Support SCI

Philanthropy, it is said, is a state of mind. But when any individual decides to give to charity, no matter how much, how do they decide who should be the recipient of their resources? Individuals are often driven through personal contact or via publicity that 'ticks their boxes'. But to support the ongoing treatment and control of schistosomiasis, that needs a special person responding to a special message.

However, SCI did have a major, unexpected new source of support, which leads me to the story of one of SCI's, and later NTD's, most generous private funding sources.

During the spring of 2006, the *Financial Times* journalist Andrew Jack contacted me about an article he was writing concerning the perceived lack of transparency in the Gates Foundation awards mechanism. He asked me to confirm his understanding that the foundation had originally funded the SCI to implement existing solutions to disease and deliver medicines to millions of people in Africa.

'Yes, that's true,' I said.

'But is it true?, he enquired, 'that with the arrival of the Foundation's new Head of Global Health, the emphasis of their granting policy has shifted from implementation to research?'

'It seems so,' I said.

He then asked if, because implementation was now outside the direct remit of the foundation, whether further funding to SCI was unlikely despite SCI's great success? Again, I had to agree with him because we had already received a message from the foundation that we would not receive further funding at the end of the current grant. What Andrew wanted to know was how did the foundation make their awards? I had no idea. He asked if I was disappointed. Of course I was disappointed, but I was not prepared to be critical of the foundation which, over six years, had been an incredibly generous and supportive donor. But I pointed out that the Gates Foundation thinking was that if we have been as success-ful as we claimed, then we should not have difficulty raising funding from other sources. So what I told the journalist, and what he quoted in his article, was that the foundation have said that they are unlikely to renew support despite the fabulously cost-effective programme we had developed which was treating millions of children at a cost of 50 US cents per child per year. Amazingly, when Andrew used this quote in his article, and said that the door was being closed by the Gates Foundation, he caused another door, fortuitously, to be opened. My quote in the article ticked a box for one of his readers. I received a call from someone the very next day, representing Sovereign Global, now known as Legatum, saying they wished to lend support to an aid project in a developing country, and were struck by the pro-poor, cost-effective figures quoted by Andrew Jack.

Naturally, I invited them to send a representative to visit us at St Mary's to learn more, and Alan McCormick, a senior executive of Sovereign, came to see me. I subjected him to a short – well, maybe not that short, but very passionate – presentation about the SCI and what we were achieving. He asked me about the needs in four specific countries and whether I would be willing to work in them: Angola, Burundi, Mozambique and Rwanda. He asked me to write a proposal for each of the countries, with work plan and budget. That sounded like a lot of work which might come to nothing so I asked him, instead, if I could prepare for him a short pre-proposal with an estimated budget for each of the countries. Sovereign Global considered what I wrote and decided to start relatively small, and they said its budget would best accommodate the health needs of Burundi, a small country with widespread STH infections, and sporadic focal schistosomiasis cases. I agreed that Burundi seemed to be the perfect 'pilot' country; and so, armed with what I perceived to be a promise, I met with the Minister of Health for Burundi at a meeting in Nairobi the following week and received her excited approval for the possibility of Burundi starting a control programme against NTDs. I explained that it would be funded by the potential donation from Alan McCormick and his financial backers.

However, I learned, on my return to London, from Alan McCormick that Sovereign Global had meanwhile changed their minds for internal reasons and decided they wanted to support Rwanda instead of Burundi. I admit that having excited the Burundi minister I felt sick at the prospect of having to go back to her to withdraw the offer of help. I explained this to Alan and, rather cheekily, suggested that instead of just supporting Rwanda for three years at a cost of just less than $5 million, why not support both countries and invest just under $10 million? After all, how cost-effective it would be to support two adjacent countries for less than $10 million. Fortunately, they were receptive and I managed to negotiate a deal which meant I left the table with more than I had bargained for: both Rwanda and Burundi received US$4.5 million to invest in a control programme for three to five years. What was a dark and gloomy cloud over the likely removal of Gates Foundation support suddenly now had a shiny silver lining thanks to Andrew Jack and the *Financial Times*, and to Alan McCormick and his colleagues at Sovereign.

I seemed to be on a run of good fortune. As we progressed to the next step, Sovereign Global told me that they wanted to run the grant through a US-based philanthropic organization known as Geneva Global. I chatted to Peter Hotez and we agreed that this was an ideal opportunity for GNNTDC to be the recipient of the grant as it would allow Geneva Global (based in the USA) to keep an eye on the administration while SCI could implement the control programmes in Burundi and Rwanda.

Meeting the Owner of Sovereign and Increasing His Investment in NTDs

Coincidentally, Geneva Global, at the time, was receiving funds from the Templeton Foundation, an organization that funds projects on science, philosophy and theology. Some weeks later, Sovereign convened a meeting in the UK in the House of Lords to honour the Templeton Foundation. I was invited to this event, and during the reception I met the chief executive and president of Sovereign/Legatum, Christopher Chandler. After we chatted he invited me to a lunch to discuss the NTD problem in Africa at greater length. Towards the end of this lunch, he asked how much would be needed to alleviate schistosomiasis across the entire sub-Saharan region of Africa.

I swiftly put together a proposal for him with a budget of $200 million a year for five years, with which I suggested we could cover the whole of sub-Saharan Africa; and I believe that Legatum (as it was by then relaunched) seriously considered it as an investment. Sadly, they did not choose to invest that much, nor add to funding SCI, because we were too specialized, I think, but they did accept the principle that they would like to support the elimination of NTDs in Africa, and they have been generous supporters of NTD control ever since. And so, Legatum donated to SCI almost $10 million to control schistosomiasis in Burundi and Rwanda and went on to do more indirectly.

The END Fund – Founded by Legatum to Raise Money from High-net-worth Individuals

In 2011, Legatum made a decision about further investment in NTDs, and instead of concentrating on schistosomiasis they aimed for an ambitious project to target all NTDs. They donated $10 million to support Geneva Global to launch a fundraising initiative named the END Fund, which was tasked with raising money from high-net-worth individuals to fight the NTD cause. The END Fund has been incredibly successful thanks to the drive of the first CEO Doug Balfour and, later, a wonderful lady, Ellen Agler, and teams led by Warren Lancaster in Europe and Ellen in the USA. SCI was, at first, the largest recipient of the funds they raised with grants going through SCI to Ethiopia, Liberia, Rwanda and Yemen. The END Fund has been very successful in raising large amounts of money, and today, Legatum implements programmes in Angola and Zimbabwe as well as supporting other NGOs like SCI.

Three examples of END Fund support are Mali, Zimbabwe and Angola. In 2012, Mali's support from USAID was abruptly curtailed after political unrest in the country and the whole USAID programme was frozen. The annual treatment against NTDs would have been lost but, fortunately, by then the END Fund had become an established supporter of NTD control and they were able to raise emergency funding to continue the annual treatment of 12 million people.

In Zimbabwe, almost all other donors were reluctant to donate because of disapproval of Robert Mugabe's misrule, but the END Fund team visited the country and funded a group of dedicated scientists who have successfully conducted MDA despite the political regime. Finally, in Angola, where language difficulties and a perception that that country did not need help had meant other donors avoided Angola, the END Fund hired a Portuguese-speaking parasitologist and funded and implemented a successful schistosomiasis control programme.

All this financial support came on the back of unprecedented donations from the pharmaceutical industry when several companies stepped in to provide their support to the NTD control movement in the form of massive drug donations. So how did all this happen and what was the result?

USAID's First Award for Integrated NTD Control and Life at RTI

It is appropriate to start with USAID because their commitment and financial contribution was the next important step, after the Gates Foundation funding, in the expansion of NTD control. Professor Peter Hotez was the person who made direct contact with influential individuals in Washington, DC, where he lived and worked at the time. In 2005, he managed to convince one or two senators to listen to the NTD story and join our lobbying campaign. Peter collaborated with Dr Eric Ottesen, Professor David Molyneux and myself to lobby Richard Green, Health Director in USAID in Washington. Our cause was helped by the fact that Richard had been my project officer during the Blue Nile Health Project when I was in Sudan, so he was familiar with NTDs. With a positive response from USAID, the four of us then reached out to Stewart Tyson, the health leader in DFID in London. Both health officers were receptive and seemingly supportive of our case, but wheels in these government departments move relatively slowly.

Eventually, USAID prepared and published a request for a proposal (known as an RFP) to fund the integration of NTD treatment programmes against at least five NTDs in several countries, with a budget of $100 million over five years. Peter, David and I collaborated to write a proposal basing the project at the Sabin Vaccine Institute, which was at the time headed by Peter. We were steaming along when we started thinking about staff and urgently needed to nominate a project director. We hoped that Eric Ottesen would agree to be nominated for the role in our submission but he was away in Fiji at the time at a meeting of the Lymphatic Filariasis Group and could not commit to take the post if we were successful.

One other component of the NTD portfolio was missing because, between us, we were lacking experience and expertise in trachoma control. To develop realistic plans for trachoma we contacted Dr Jacob Kumaresan, the then director of the International Trachoma Institute (ITI), and he agreed to join our consortium. He did, however, suggest that he would feel happier joining us if our proposal was not through the relatively small and inexperienced Sabin Institute. He recommended that we would be more likely to win the bid if we went under the umbrella of an established USA contractor because of the size of the award. The best available contractor was the Research Triangle Institute (RTI), so we asked them to front the bid, which they agreed to do. They, however, had no one qualified for the project director position, and so even though I was Director of SCI at the time, I agreed to be nominated. Our bid was successful, but things did not turn out quite as we, the authors of the bid, had imagined. RTI insisted that, as they were now the award holders, the secretariat could not be housed at the Sabin Institute but had to be situated and staffed at RTI. Sadly, Peter and I had no choice but to accept this ultimatum, but this meant I had to take a leave of absence from SCI and Imperial College and be employed as an RTI employee.

In the proposal to USAID we had proposed building on the SCI programmes in Burkina Faso, Mali, Niger and Uganda, adding in Ghana and Sierra Leone as new countries. The prime contractor, RTI, could sub-contract SCI to implement the expanded programmes in Niger, Burkina Faso and Uganda, ensuring that the programmes initially funded by the Gates Foundation would continue in these three countries until at least 2011. USAID funds would also pass through RTI to Mali and Ghana with both programmes managed by ITI, and to Sierra Leone, which would be managed by Helen Keller International.

During the initial phase as director, I travelled extensively for six months setting up the programmes in the countries and talking to USAID offices in each country before approaching the ministries of health. In Washington we had to arrange the contractual bureaucracy before we could transfer funding via RTI and their sub-contractors to the countries.

With the idea of a possible long-term appointment, Margie and I looked at properties in DC. However, I was convinced that, ideally, I would manage the project from the UK rather than move to DC, because I envisaged a lot of travel to the countries, and so from Washington I would have two overnight flights to reach any of the recipient countries, whereas I could reach any country from London in one day or night, and could also return to DC, if needed, within a few hours. Sadly, this proposal did not meet with the approval of RTI nor with the USAID's new health staff, Irene Koch and Christie Hanson.

That was a real learning curve for me and I stuck it out for six months, but with much less authority than I had envisaged. I had employees imposed on me by senior management and I could not travel to the African countries without approval from some hidden senior, nameless persons in the hierarchy of RTI. In addition, my every move was closely subjected to scrutiny and approval from the two staffers at USAID. When I was called into USAID and told that my continuation as director depended on my moving to Washington and being ever-present at the RTI office, I made the difficult decision to quit the directorship and move back to the UK and to SCI. However, no one is indispensable, and without me the RTI management of the USAID funding has been very successful, and much more funding has passed to them over the years so that RTI and USAID can be incredibly proud of how they have taken NTDs to the verge of elimination in many countries.

A New Concept - Rapid Impact Package - Introduced

A treatment strategy known as the Rapid Impact Package was developed by the GNNTDC group with Dr Lorenzo Savioli and Dr Dirk Engels (NTD Department at WHO, Geneva). The network had advocated, with the WHO NTD team, the adoption of an integrated treatment of the seven major NTDs with a combination of donated drugs.

These drugs were albendazole (GSK) or mebendazole (Johnson & Johnson) for STH; albendazole and Mectizan (Merck USA) for lymphatic filariasis in Africa; albendazole and diethylcarbamazine (DEC) for LF outside of Africa; ivermectin (Merck) for onchocerciasis; praziquantel (Merck KGaA, formally E. Merck) for schistosomiasis and azithromycin (Pfizer) for trachoma.

At the time GNNTDC was launched, some of these drugs were being donated by large pharmaceutical companies, but not yet in the quantities required to expand to national coverage in all the endemic countries. Merck and GSK were committed to meeting the need against LF and onchocerciasis, but GSK did not donate albendazole for STH until the 2010 WHO Partnership for Parasite Control meeting when Andrew Witty (then CEO of GSK, now *Sir* Andrew Witty) committed to the donation of even more albendazole to de-worm school-age children. From 2010, GSK donated 1 billion tablets of albendazole per annum.

The early donation of praziquantel by MedPharm (a drug distributor) had stopped by 2007 but was replaced, fortuitously, by a new donation provided by E. Merck (also known as Merck Serono and, latterly, as Merck KGaA). As for the other NTDs, Pfizer had joined the donors in 1999 by providing azithromycin through the International Trachoma Initiative for treatment of trachoma, and their donation increased as more and more trachoma country programmes started.

Johnson & Johnson is another company donating against NTDs with their drug mebendazole – which is better than albendazole against ascariasis – with 50 million tablets a year in 2007 and increasing to 200 million tablets a year in 2010.

These donations were instrumental to the successful acceptance of the concept of the Rapid Impact Package (more about this in Chapter 19). They were also instrumental in realizing the integration of the timing of delivery of the different treatments and achieving the average cost of US 50 cents per person p.a. As time has gone by, integration has come to mean collaboration, co-operation and communication to ensure optimum timing of delivery, rather than emphasizing the delivery of all the package of drugs at one visit.

The Wheel of Fortune Is Spun for NTDs

From 2007 to 2015, NTDs rose rapidly up the donor agenda, urged on by more frequent references in peer-reviewed publications (demonstrating successful control), and by international bodies and globally supported declarations, including by Bill Gates himself. Furthermore, the MDGs aimed at halving world poverty by 2015 gave credence to the fight against NTDs, and the Director General of WHO, Dr Margaret Chan, regularly made a point of publicly supporting NTD control efforts and highlighting the issue far more than previous administrations had done. The clear attraction of investing resources in NTDs, which was brought to the attention of various authorities, is that they promise workable solutions and measurable changes in morbidity over the next decade with immediate, discernable improvements after treatment. The prospect of elimination of these diseases by 2020 became the first ambitious goal, but when all partners realized that the resources to reach that goal did not exist, that target date was soon changed to 2030.

SCI collaborates with COR in Atlanta

In a way, the Centre for Operational Research for Neglected Tropical Diseases (COR-NTDs), based at the Task Force for Global Health in Atlanta, took over the mantle of advocacy and communication from the GNNTDC. COR-NTDs received substantial financial support from both USAID, DFID and the Gates Foundation, and was co-directed by the strong partnership of Dr Patrick Lammie and Dr Eric Ottesen. Its role was to fill in gaps in research which would support specific NTD programmes and highlight synergies between the programmes.

A particularly valuable contribution for all global NTD researchers and implementers was their organization of a three-day annual meeting of the NTD community. These meetings were convened either before or after, but at the same venue as, the American Society of Tropical Medicine and Hygiene annual November meetings. As such, the meetings were held in Atlanta, Philadelphia, Baltimore, New Orleans and Washington, DC, depending on the ASTMH venue. In the early days of these meetings, when they followed the ASTMH (2002–2006), perhaps 20–30 people attended, but by 2012 and beyond there were 500 people interested and involved in NTD research and control attending the new COR meetings. One of the regular attenders at these meetings was Dr Dominique Kyelem, a scientist from Burkina Faso who worked with SCI, and was Programme Director for Neglected Tropical Diseases at the Task Force for Global Health in Atlanta. Sadly, he suffered from cancer, and after battling the illness, he died, aged just 51, in 2013 (see his memorial at end of this book).

Three Special Meetings of ASTMH/COR

Matchmaker Margie, make us a match

It is 2008. An ASTMH meeting/dinner was held in honour of Narcis Kabatereine for all his work and long-serving support. The SCI team were well represented. To that meeting we had invited Narcis' partner, Peace, at SCI's expense. One evening, when the SCI team members were at a jazz club, my wife Margie sat next to Peace and casually asked her whether she and Narcis had ever contemplated marriage. The story Peace told her was that she and Narcis had dated when she was 17 years of age and still at school. Narcis had proposed but Peace said no because she wanted to finish her education and open her own business. Narcis, being several years older than Peace, moved on and married someone else and raised a family. Sadly, his first wife died, and later his friends tried to fix him up with another. Not knowing the history between them, one friend invited Peace and Narcis to dinner. They immediately hit it off, and as Peace had never married, they 'hooked up', but did not marry. Margie asked Peace if that bothered her and Peace said she really did want to get married, even though they would not have children. So Margie, being Margie, tackled Narcis and became their 'matchmaker'. Narcis agreed to propose to Peace but only on the condition that if she accepted, Margie and I would fly to Kampala to be the guests of honour at their wedding. Well, of course, we agreed.

When a date was finally set for the wedding, it was not at a period when we could take much time off, so our trip to Kampala would be a bit of a 'whistle-stop tour'. We flew to Entebbe on Friday 8 December 2009, arriving at about midnight and staying that night at a nearby airport hotel. The next morning we took a taxi into Kampala and went straight to the church for the wedding. The reception was amazing and because there were 600 people attending it was held in the grounds of a school. The guests were grouped in tents – one tent for special guests (including us), one tent for Narcis' workplace members (Ministry of Health), one tent each for Peace's and Narcis' home villagers, and at least two other tents besides.

We were due to fly back to London the following day, so we had booked into the Serena Hotel for one night only and Narcis and Peace spent their wedding night in the same hotel. The four of us were therefore able to spend a very friendly day together on the Sunday before we flew home. We arrived back in the UK at 6 am on Monday morning – tired but very happy that all had gone so well.

ASTMH Award 2012

In 2012 I was awarded the title of Honorary Member of the ASTMH. Every year, ASTMH awarded honorary membership to four non-American scientists. I was one of the four, together with Aldo Lima from Brazil; Kevin Marsh, a British malariologist based in Kenya; and Marcel Tanner, Director of the Swiss Tropical Institute.

Dominique Kyelem Prize 2018

In 2018 I was awarded the Dominique Kyelem Prize, a prize honouring the Burkina Faso scientist credited with fantastic work in eliminating LF.

Harnessing the Power of Big Pharma to Support Our Programmes

Large pharmaceutical companies and bad press tend to go hand in hand. No matter what efforts are made to promote and publish stories attesting to positive corporate or social responsibility, there will always be a plethora of stories and rumours to discredit this profitable industry. Nobody doubts that pharma has profits as their driver, but each company also has a large staff who wish to work for a caring and responsible company. Their scientists take pleasure in seeing their discoveries put to good use. Shareholders also, increasingly, wish to see that they have invested in ethical companies. Indeed, George Merck, the founder of the drug company bearing his name, is quoted as saying to his shareholders: 'We try never to forget medicine is for people not for profits'; and after gasps of surprise from those gathered, he then added, 'but we know that the profits will follow'.

So it is that often the good news emanating from the pharma community can be lost in the murky telling of the bad – news such as the significant altruistic contributions they have made to the war on the diseases I have been outlining in this book and which I summarize below:

- **Merck USA** (Merck Sharp Dome), a company in the USA, has donated ivermectin to treat onchocerciasis (river blindness) since 1986 and LF since 1996.
- **Pfizer** started donating azithromycin for trachoma in 1999.
- **GSK** donated albendazole for LF from 1999, but then in 2010, they expanded their commitment, and increased their albendazole donation to treat STH.
- **Merck KGaA,** a German company, agreed to donate some praziquantel against schistosomiasis and then incrementally increased their donation to 100 million doses per year.
- **Johnson & Johnson** provide mebendazole, also for STH.

These five companies fund all costs associated with manufacture, packaging and shipping to the port of the destination country. After arrival, costs are usually met by the government of the recipient country, either from its own resources or from bilateral aid, or charity or NGO donations.

These drugs, currently donated to treat diseases in the poorest countries, were developed many decades ago but, despite use in the developed world for both human and veterinarian treatments, had mostly been unavailable in Africa prior to 2000 (except for Mectizan against onchocerciasis). For example, albendazole was marketed as a veterinary product, and profits from this market offset many of the costs relating to research and development for human use. Corporate responsibility has increased exponentially since the millennium, and the companies which have made profits from these medications are now giving back to the poor people who cannot afford to buy their products.

Drug donations are, of course, very well received and have revolutionized the treatment of tropical diseases in the world's poorest countries. However, donations need to be fed into programmes that are sustainable and into country health systems that can distribute products responsibly and safely. Fortunately, most countries have risen to the challenge and taken advantage of the generous donations. They all now have ongoing control programmes, thanks to the efforts of the WHO, supported, respectively, by the USAID-funded RTI; the African Programme for Onchocerciasis Control (APOC); the Liverpool School of Tropical Medicine Lymphatic Filariasis Support Programme (GAELF, now the Centre for Neglected Tropical Diseases); the International Trachoma Initiative (ITI); and the SCI, to name a few. Other organizations involved with implementation include Sightsavers, Helen Keller International (HKI), the END Fund, and Health Development International (HDI).

Merck, Mectizan and the fight against river blindness

In 1985, William C. Campbell at Merck and Satoshi Ōmura in Japan discovered a novel therapy against infections caused by roundworm parasites.

Ivermectin (Mectizan) was originally used for the treatment of worms in horses and dogs, but after conducting a seven-year-long clinical trial in Africa, with the support of the WHO, it was shown that an annual dose of ivermectin would sterilize onchocerca worms. This sterilization not only helped to break transmission via the blackfly but also, because no larvae were produced by the sterile adults, people no longer suffered from the severe itching and the irreversible blindness the larvae caused. The incumbent CEO of Merck, Roy Vagelos, realized that although the drug had fantastic potential for improving the quality of life for millions of West Africans, it was not available to the residents of rural African countries because of their poverty. He therefore committed his company to supplying the drug free of charge to prevent onchocerciasis (river blindness) until blindness was eliminated.

In 1960, an estimated 40% of people aged 40 and above living near rivers in West Africa were blind. Since 1985, the Merck-donated Mectizan now reaches over 70 million people annually in 35 countries in Africa and South America. Who knows how much the donation has so far cost the company? But it is safe to say that millions of people who would be blind are now living on the banks of rivers without an onchocerciasis infection. Merck has deservedly gained a massive benefit in good publicity as people have come to appreciate their donation, not to mention that river blindness has been eliminated in most South American countries, and has been all but eliminated in sub-Saharan Africa. Thirty years after this ground-breaking discovery, William Campbell and Satoshi Omura (both in their eighties) were awarded a Nobel Prize in 2015 for their work and the benefits that ivermectin has brought to millions of people in Africa. This was an unexpected award, and an honour felt by the NTD community. Then, four years later, it was followed by another award, because in 2019 the Nobel Prize for Economics was awarded to Michael Kremer for his work calculating the benefits of de-worming.

E-Merck and praziquantel

In 2007, the European company E-Merck (aka Merck Serono/Merck KGaA) decided to donate 20 million praziquantel tablets a year to WHO; enough to treat around 8 million children. This was a relatively small percentage of the need, but WHO used the donation to encourage a few countries to start a control initiative. In response to the explanation of the need of children in Africa, in 2012 Merck announced they would provide an incremental expansion of their commitment, and in 2015 they had donated 105 million tablets. By 2018 they reached their target and donated 250 million tablets, which was enough to treat 100 million school-age children; and, furthermore, this donation would continue until it was no longer needed.

A lesson learned – scale up development and healthcare together

The most poignant lesson we learnt in building partnerships, which is becoming increasingly evident as NTD control programmes scale up, is that to be effective healthcare and international development agendas around the world need to scale up in parallel. The tools to alleviate much of the misery of the poorest of the poor already exist in one form or another, but they will not deliver themselves. What makes the challenge presented by NTDs so much more manageable is simply that we use safe treatments, which need to be delivered just once a year. The solution now lies in harnessing and synergizing the strengths of different partners – from those that tread the luxurious red carpets in the House of Lords in London to teachers and children in their mud-walled school houses, which bake under the equatorial sun.

16 The SCI Target – Low Infection Rates

The World Health Organization has developed guidelines to advise national ministries on how best to tackle schistosomiasis using MDA as its main tool. Determining how often to administer treatment and to whom depends on the level of infection in the community. In the past, because of limited resources (including praziquantel availability), each national government was encouraged to develop their programme to find the balance between treatment frequency and the use and cost of a scarce drug.

Moving to Elimination – A Mixed Bag

Getting to and maintaining low infection rates are prerequisites to moving towards the elimination of the disease. The number of countries supported by SCI did not change from the original six until after 2006. Thereafter, more countries were added after funding by the USAID, two more countries through Legatum's private donation and then even more countries were added when DFID started their NTD programme support in 2010.

This meant that although 14 countries were treating their inhabitants in 2014, maybe 25 countries had still to start with disease (morbidity) control, while some of the earlier supported countries were ready to move towards elimination, meaning that there were no new cases appearing. Continuous control measures since 2003 have meant that lower prevalence and transmission rates have already been reached in several countries, especially those peripheral to the highly endemic areas of Africa.

Globally, in 2012, schistosomiasis in Puerto Rico, Morocco, Oman, Mauritius and some of the Caribbean islands was near elimination. The success was probably due to the fact that climatic conditions meant transmission was only seasonal and a variety of control measures had been successfully applied over the years including chemotherapy (treatment with drugs), snail control and sanitation. Puerto Rico was an example of socio-economic development leading to better hygiene and reduced water contact interrupting transmission.

A well-managed programme in Morocco reduced prevalence of *S. haematobium* from 10,645 cases in 1983 to 231 cases in 1999. By 2003, there were a mere handful of cases in the Tala province and the disease is now deemed to have achieved elimination.

In 2005, in most countries, lymphatic filariasis, yaws and trachoma were considered as targets for elimination and even eradication, because of the tools available (including donated drugs) and financial support. Schistosomiasis was not considered to be a disease targeted for eradication or, even more realistically, elimination. However, by the time of the May 2012 World Health Assembly (WHA), African ministers of health accepted an ambitious resolution calling for all countries *to work towards* elimination of schistosomiasis but recognizing that only in some countries, or parts of them, was elimination beginning to appear as a possibility.

Saudi Arabia, in 2012 Down to 1% and Now ...

Saudi Arabia provides an example, referenced by the WHA, of the successful interplay of these different factors. By 2012, both *S. haematobium* and *S. mansoni* were endemic at levels of only 1% prevalence, down from focal levels of 40% in 1980, because of a control strategy implemented since 1985 using chemotherapy, mollusciciding in appropriate areas, and health education. The success was, in part, due to the integration of control measures, but also because the government invested in integrated schistosomiasis control efforts within the primary healthcare system, which had greater than 90% coverage.

Unlike in sub-Saharan Africa, 95% of the Saudi population have access to potable water and most children attend school. However, migration and immigration of infected people from neighbouring areas continue to present a risk of disease re-emergence. Today, half of those individuals with schistosomiasis in Saudi Arabia are immigrants, and the question remains: will they contribute to ongoing transmission?

WHO Dual Strategy for Control and Elimination of Schistosomiasis

Following the WHA resolution of 2012, the WHO developed a dual strategy for the control and elimination of schistosomiasis. Thus, in a high-burden country, the ministry of health should implement a strategy for morbidity control adapted to the public health context. In areas where a low endemic level has been reached and elimination may be feasible, the strategy is to consolidate control and move to elimination. This dual strategy was incorporated into a 'road map for elimination by 2020', an ambitious goal that has not been achieved globally; 2030 is now the target for many countries. The Gates Foundation has taken the initiative to annually record the milestones for achieving the road map, not only for schistosomiasis but also for all the NTDs in the WHO list. Based at Sightsavers, the project is named 'Uniting to Combat NTDs', and collects data on each NTD as the countries progress to elimination.

What Is the Likelihood of Elimination?

In determining the likelihood that schistosomiasis in any country in sub-Saharan Africa can be eliminated, we must take on board the fact that schistosomiasis has a complex transmission cycle and in many individuals is largely asymptomatic. Less definitive is the role that animal reservoirs may play in the life cycle of *S. mansoni*.

These make a WHO definition of criteria, and therefore certification for elimination, a difficult issue. To confidently declare that transmission has been interrupted depends on specialists making a detailed assessment of the risk of re-emergence or re-introduction, even on a focal level.

The degree of certainty that no new cases have been infected also depends very much on the sensitivity of the surveillance system and, in particular, the sensitivity of the diagnostic method used for evaluation (Engels *et al.*, 2002). The circulating cathodic antigen (CCA) urine-cassette assay is more sensitive than Kato-Katz smears. A study (in which SCI took part) among 500 schoolchildren in Uganda showed the CCA to be a good survey tool for *Schistosoma mansoni* in areas where the disease is declining (Adriko *et al.*, 2014).

Testing the hypothesis

In countries where the disease target was that schistosomiasis be deemed 'no longer a public health problem', MDA was not enough and sustainable transmission control was required. This would depend on the provision, or improvement, of hygiene and sanitation; and environmental management, where possible, should become a major operational target.

Ongoing surveillance should monitor the risk of resurgence of schistosomiasis. Egypt was the country where I hoped to demonstrate that this hypothesis was correct, and yes, we were successful. When I left in 2002, the country was well along the way to complete elimination having eliminated the public health problem and reduced prevalence to below 2%.

Sadly, the Arab Spring uprising in Egypt and the overthrow of President Mubarak in 2011 caused political upheaval and delayed any additional elimination efforts. This situation has highlighted just how important good governance and political stability are to disease control in general and schistosomiasis in particular.

A significant discussion point is around a phrase used earlier – 'schistosomiasis no longer a public health problem'. This phrase has been used in WHO publications and in many papers by various authors to be the first target of a control programme. But what does this mean? And did SCI's MDA strategy at minimized cost reach our target? And was schistosomiasis 'no longer a public health problem' in the first six countries we tackled?

Is it, in fact, a scientifically definable target?

There are several scientific and technical advisory groups (STAGs) with scientists from all over the globe who meet annually to make technical recommendations to WHO, and one of them is focused on NTDs. Some members of the NTD-STAG at the time I was on the committee have spoken out against the use of this phrase 'no longer a public health problem' as they argue it cannot be accurately defined.

The NTD-STAG, established in 2010 by Dr Lorenzo Savioli, the Director of the NTD department, has become an important annual forum for discussion of progress towards global coverage and advising WHO on policy. I was thrilled to be invited to join the advisory group, which consisted of about 15 scientific advisors, representatives from the various regions of WHO, members of the NTD department (as observers) and some NGOs and donors (also as observers). In addition, expert sub-committees meet regularly to discuss different aspects of NTDs, which includes the preparation of a booklet on methodologies for interventions.

Now there is another coincidence (and a link back to Arusha, Tanzania). The current NTD department director is one Dr Mwele Malecela.

Mwele, and 'Alan's Not the Vicar'

During the time I lived in Arusha, the East African Community was formed, with its headquarters in Arusha. The three countries, Kenya, Uganda and Tanzania, were at their most co-operative and friends in 1968. The Minister to the EAC from Tanzania was John Malacela and he and his wife Ezerina and their children lived next door to Irene and me in Barabara ya Serengeti. John and Ezerina had a child in Arusha soon after their arrival but that child sadly died at a very young age and my then wife Irene played the organ in church for the funeral which I attended as a neighbour. The vicar (who was similar in build to me) and I were the only white people at the funeral and a few days later when I met John outside his house he said, 'Oh, yes, you are the vicar.' I said, 'No John, the vicar was the other white man at the funeral and I am your neighbour', at which John said, 'Sorry, but I cannot always tell you white people apart', which made me laugh.

We got to know John and Ezerina quite well and they threw a party in their garden for our daughter Janet's christening in 1969. Their six-year-old daughter Mwele was there at the feast. When I met Mwele some 20 years later at a tropical medicine conference event in Washington, DC, to celebrate the 100th anniversary of the London School of Hygiene and Tropical Medicine, I introduced myself and reminded her of our 'history'. 'Yes,' she said, 'I still have a photo on my bedside table of me at the age of six cradling a newborn white baby – your baby Janet.'

Mwele rose to be the Director of the Medical Research Institute in Tanzania, and was the driving force behind the speedily expanded programme to eliminate LF in Tanzania. She then joined WHO in 2015. John himself had a magnificent career becoming Prime Minister of Tanzania.

17 Research – Forewarned is Forearmed

Recruitment of a New Deputy Director of SCI, 2009

In 2007, when both I and Howard Thompson reached the age of 65, Howard kindly retired, allowing me the opportunity to recruit a new Deputy Director young enough to be the one who would eventually take over the reins at SCI. Professor David Molyneux recommended Dr Wendy Harrison, a trained veterinarian who had experience of working in the USA, Rwanda and Uganda, and with GSK in UK.

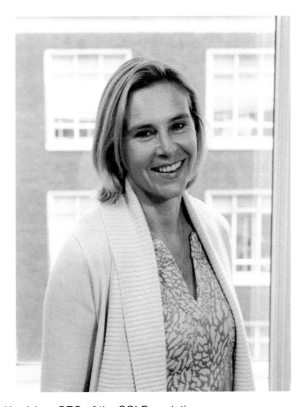

Fig. 17.1. Wendy Harrision, CEO of the SCI Foundation.

© Fenwick, Norris and McCall 2022. *A Tale of a Man, a Worm and a Snail: The Schistosomiasis Control Initiative* (A. Fenwick *et al.*)
DOI: 10.1079/9781786392558.0017

We advertised the post and interviewed several candidates. By the time we worked our way through the Imperial recruitment process and selected Wendy, it was March 2009 before she joined.

Wendy and I worked in the same room for nine years, which bordered on sainthood on her part, but she stuck it out and did eventually take over from me. One of the new aspects of epidemiology that Wendy brought to SCI was her interest in the synergy between animal and human public health and how neatly schistosomiasis fits into this. Her field experience was to prove very useful.

During the years that we worked together, Wendy showed a very useful talent for administration and for motivating the staff who were programme managers.

And as the time for me to retire approached, she started planning her promotion and brought experts in to define the structure of SCI going forward (mentioned in Chapter 20). Since my handover, as Director of SCI she has led the organization to even greater visibility, with SCI eventually striking out away from Imperial College, as an independent charity named SCI Foundation.

Key Operational Questions Remaining in 2009

As Wendy joined, there were a number of operational research questions facing the team. Was it all too good to be true? Could the treatment with albendazole and praziquantel costing just US$0.50 per person, per year, control two parasitic diseases, and possibly lead to their elimination as a public health problem?

Could the immediate benefits and the long-term benefits to children receiving the treatment be proved? And then some really important research questions were: How many treatments does it take to protect a child into adulthood? Can treated children develop any resistance to further infection? Can we move into 'praziquantel holidays' – that is treating every two years instead of annually – and when can we safely stop treatments?

Most serious were the questions: Will over-use of praziquantel result in the development of drug resistance among the parasite population? If resistance develops, will the benefits of disease control reaped so far by the SCI be lost to future generations? Does drug pressure change the parasite and, if so, in which way? What are these hotspots that seem to be stubbornly difficult in making reductions in prevalence? What other unpredictable negative consequences will appear?

Thus, there were in 2009 some key operational research questions which needed to be addressed by the SCI monitoring and evaluation team in parallel with our implementation and expanding treatment coverage. The hope was that the answers would show that long-term control of schistosomiasis is worthwhile. Indeed, the long-term goal will be elimination in many parts of Africa; but will that be reached, and if so by when?

2030 is still a worthwhile target. By 2019, when the SCI left the umbrella of Imperial College to launch as an independent charity, over 200 million treatments had been delivered with SCI assistance and the foundation's annual budget would be £20 million.

Research Gaps: The Knowns and the Unknowns

There are other gaps in our knowledge of schistosomiasis which SCI cannot address. One is the hope that one day the groups searching for a vaccine will be successful.

This chapter now focuses on those research questions which link most directly to the work of the SCI and what our research team have discovered about the interactions in Africa between human host and schistosome parasite.

The programme managers at the SCI mainly focus on implementation while the research scientists, led by Professor Joanne Webster, develop studies to investigate issues directly linked to maintaining public health in sub-Saharan Africa. On a more academic level, however, Joanne developed associations with other parasitologists to actively investigate issues such as drug resistance and ways that the worms interact with the human immune system. SCI has not worked in isolation, and so to add further depth and context we refer to some key work within the wider field of schistosome research, and include our collaborators Professor David Rollinson, Bonnie Webster and Fiona Allan at the Natural History Museum and, more recently, the SCORE team based at the University of Georgia in Athens, Georgia. We also have been grateful for the collaboration of many African research scientists working in their own countries.

To be more successful, research into schistosomiasis and schistosomes should be a collaborative exercise across several countries and institutions. Each incremental addition to the pool of available data adds to overall understanding of the parasite, the disease and methods of control.

Keeping One Step Ahead of Resistance

There are many examples of resistance developing because of wide-scale use of drugs or agents against a particular species of organism. Malaria is an excellent example where drugs such as chloroquine and paludrin are no longer effective for treating cases of malaria in humans, and where one insecticide after another no longer kills mosquitoes. If the parasite, bacteria or virus has high genetic variability, then certain gene combinations are more likely to have a constitution which resists the effects of each drug. These organisms may then survive the treatment against them whilst others (which are susceptible) die. With the majority of organisms culled by the widespread use of a single drug, resistant survivors will thrive and dominate the remaining population and the next generations.

At this point, drug intervention becomes less effective and eventually that drug will no longer have a lethal effect, and a state of drug resistance has emerged. At that point the drug has no future. Without any intervention to control reproduction, growth and therefore transmission, the resistant parasite, bacteria or virus can multiply and freely infect the host population.

Praziquantel dosage

Praziquantel is still the *only* drug in use in the battle against schistosomiasis and has been so since 1980. Several different dosage regimes were tested including two doses of 20 mg/kg body weight, the first given after breakfast and the second given after lunch on the same day. This was thought likely to reduce unpleasant side-effects. However, after many trials, praziquantel is now administered at a recommended single dose of 40 mg/kg of body weight given after any meal; this has been proven as equally effective for treating all the major schistosome species, *S. japonicum*, *S. mansoni* and *S. haematobium*.

Confusing cure rates

Rather confusingly, reports by different researchers in different endemic situations have claimed cure rates which varied between 60% and 90% with different criteria and methods selected. Thus, each evaluation should define the parasite species, the pre-treatment intensity of infection in each individual treated, and then the timing and number of the post-treatment follow-up examinations. Occasionally, situations arose where praziquantel appeared to be 'ineffective' because 'cure rates' were low 12 months after the treatment – but there are alternative explanations for the lower than expected 'cure rate'. The first is that in heavy infections there are many worms in the host's body pre-treatment and, inevitably, some of them survive and continue to lay eggs; the second is when the treated population includes individuals harbouring immature worms. Praziquantel does not kill the immature stages of the schistosomes, and therefore after treatment, the immature worms continue to maturity and start laying eggs.

A third possibility is that the human populations living in areas of high transmission rapidly becoming re-infected in the months after treatment and so at the 12-month follow-up examinations, re-infections have appeared, and maybe this has been considered to be a drug failure.

In my opinion, there is little evidence to date to suggest that the cure rates have changed in natural populations and I believe, perhaps as an optimist, that no resistance has developed.

Belief in praziquantel

I believe that praziquantel is as good as it gets. Mostly, the drug is effective and there are few side-effects suffered by those who are treated, and they are mild and transient effects observed in a small proportion of patients. Toxicity and serious side-effects are negligible. Other transient side-effects include stomach pains. These are strongly correlated with the intensity of infection and are believed to result from a flood of breakdown products released from the bodies of dying schistosomes.

However, we are aware that the 600 mg praziquantel tablets are not perfect for young children. The tablet has a bitter taste and so a child biting into the tablet instead of swallowing it whole may vomit. Because of this, and the growing realization that schistosomiasis is an important disease if contracted by infants, a consortium led by Merck has been working for several years to produce a formulation of praziquantel which will be palatable for children (a paediatric praziquantel).

Why I believe resistance is a minimal threat

The facts

In villages in the Nile Delta region of Egypt, a few cases of treatment failure were recorded and reduced parasite sensitivity to praziquantel was confirmed in the laboratory. The worms which had survived the treatment were bred in the laboratory from the eggs taken from the uncured patients. However, the level of reduced killing power by praziquantel was relatively small and nowhere near the level at which it could be classed as resistance (Ismail *et al.*, 1996; 1999).

What was later shown in the laboratory and in follow-up studies in the Egyptian villages was that these genotypes, which are potentially resistant to praziquantel, have apparently not spread and treatment has continued to be highly efficacious in the Nile Delta even after ten years of annual intervention.

The findings from Egypt suggest praziquantel resistance does not appear to pose an obvious or immediate threat to the success of the treatment programmes. In northern Senegal, in the 1980s, initial reports of low clearance rates during mass treatment raised concerns over resistance (Brown, 1994), but reviews of laboratory studies have since eliminated this as the main cause of apparent treatment failure (Danso-Appiah and De Vlas, 2002; Gryseels *et al.*, 2001). The Senegal data satisfies me that the apparent failure of praziquantel in that country reflected a special epidemiological situation of very high endemicity and not resistance (see Chapter 9; dam construction and loss of crayfish predator of snails).

Other scientists have suggested that there are scientific reasons to believe that praziquantel-based resistance has not become an issue in natural populations so far (Doenhoff and Pica-Mattoccia, 2006), although some isolated reports of possible resistance have been documented (Ribeiro dos Santos *et al.*, 2006).

Since 1990, several hundred millions of treatments have been delivered in over 20 countries, and the general impression is that resistance, while always possible, is some way off, and indeed may never happen.

There are three main reasons behind why I believe resistance is not a threat.

The first is that the laboratory-bred worms which have been found to need a higher dose of praziquantel to kill them have proved to be weak in terms of reproduction; in addition, the fact that the relevant gene which confers resistance is recessive and therefore less likely to develop.

The second is that there is almost always 'refugia' in the treated areas, meaning that the coverage of treatment is usually well below 100% of the population, in which case some non-resistant worms will survive in the environment along with any potential resistant worms, and thus any resistant strains which may have developed will be diluted by susceptible strains.

A third factor that hinders the development of resistance is the very long time it takes to complete the life cycle from adult worms pairing up in the human liver to complete the cycle to the next generation. The life cycle and turnover of parasites is slow compared to parasites like malaria, which reproduce on a daily basis. Schistosomes live anything from three to 20 years so the chance for interbreeding between resistant parasites is low.

As a reminder of their complex life cycle, it takes two months from an adult female schistosome worm laying an egg to the next generation of female worm laying her egg. The cycle takes two months because the egg has to pass into the bladder or intestine to be excreted into water; then it must hatch into miracidia, which infect a snail. Inside the snail, asexual reproduction process takes a month – each miracidium changes into a sporocyst, which in turn generates more sporocysts, before cercaria emerge from the snail and infect back to the human – and then another month for the schistosomule to develop into an adult worm laying eggs.

A final related factor is that this is a large worm and therefore complicated in constitution.

Farmers use *refugia* to prevent development of resistance in cattle against worms

The treatment of worms in cattle illustrates the principle of *refugia*. When farmers treat a field of worm-infested cattle with any anthelminthic drug, they treat every single cow. Thus, the only living worms that are likely to survive this 100% coverage in the cows are those with at least some propensity for resistance.

If all surviving worms in a field are resistant to some degree, then they will breed to produce resistant offspring. To counteract this effect, farmers use the principle of *refugia* during treatment campaigns. This means leaving some of the cows in a field untreated, thus mixing treated with untreated animals, and so diluting the effect of resistance in that herd. By purposely providing a pool of susceptible genes, the resistant genes in the population are diluted with some susceptible ones. In this way, the likelihood that resistance will develop depends on the proportion of the parasite population in *refugia* during treatment. For example, in eastern Ethiopia, farmers were able to reverse high levels of multi-drug resistance to a variety of de-worming drugs in a flock of goats by introducing mixed grazing with a sheep flock that did not show resistance.

In human mass-chemotherapy treatment programmes, because we rarely treat 100% of the population, *refugia* is naturally present. This is assisted by the fact that the selective pressure is low because praziquantel is short-acting and only given annually. We only realistically aim for 75% coverage of the population, and so in highly endemic areas there are still many untreated individuals who are either absent or avoid or even refuse to take the treatment. Other reservoirs of untreated parasites at the time of the MDA are, first, infected snail hosts shedding cercariae, and second, immature worms which are not susceptible to the action of praziquantel.

Potential for praziquantel resistance from worm genetics

The innate ability of all organisms (including schistosomes) to alter their make-up so they become resistant to a drug involves a change in their genome. Such an evolutionary change in response to drug therapy may be predicted as a possibility since schistosomes have been shown to have sufficient genetic variability to evolve and co-evolve (Davies *et al.*, 2002; Gower and Webster, 2005; Webster and Davies, 2001; Webster *et al.*, 2007; Woolhouse *et al.*, 2002).

Also, using artificial selection culture techniques in the laboratory, a low level of praziquantel resistance in *S. mansoni* has been demonstrated within as few as six generations (Fallon and Doenhoff, 1994). Albeit that these findings were in an artificial environment, there is still cause for concern because they have illustrated the potential for resistance to praziquantel. Furthermore, combined with a known praziquantel efficacy of less than 90% (Mutapi *et al.*, 1998) and the intensive and prolonged selection pressures that are being imposed by MDA programmes, one might assume that the potential for praziquantel resistance developing and/or spreading within the natural setting is not negligible. We must not be complacent, so continuous vigilance is needed. Finding practical methods to track any development of drug resistance is therefore a key area of schistosome research.

But, even within China, where praziquantel has been successfully used widely for over 30 years, no evidence has been found to suggest the development of resistance.

SCI Operational Research – Impact Studies on Our Programmes

Operational research at SCI is conducted as part of our M&E activities to demonstrate the impact of the programmes. I have already stressed how important it is to demonstrate to donors (particularly DFID) and to implementing governments that the treatment interventions result in a significant reduction in infection rates, morbidity, disease prevalence and intensity of infection.

The operational research team is currently headed by Dr Fiona Fleming, a long-term staff member of SCI. Fiona was one of the first to join SCI having started as a programme manager for Zambia and Uganda, but who successfully completed and defended her PhD on the cost and cost benefits of treatment before being promoted to the position of Director of Monitoring, Evaluation and Research.

From 2003 to 2019, several impact studies have been completed and published by SCI staff. One early example is from three primary schools from the Mayuge district in Uganda, which have provided detailed longitudinal data on infection intensities and prevalence (Kabatereine *et al.*, 2007). The findings were as follows.

At each of three follow-up studies, at six months, one year and two years post-treatment with praziquantel, the intensity of infection had been driven down dramatically. Even in those children who were 'not completely cured', either because of re-infection or some surviving worms, still their egg output showed a reduced infection intensity, and egg output rarely, if ever, returned to pre-treatment levels.

What was very promising was that the percentage of children getting re-infected also dropped over time. The worrying downside to the results was that some children were positive at each return visit. Individuals who were more heavily infected before treatment were found to be more likely to be positive at follow-up; possibly they had experienced re-infection. This predisposition could be due to genetic or immune responses but may also be due to the child's water-contact behaviour.

But there are other factors which may be affecting our results and interpretation of these results. Firstly, current methods of monitoring cure rates and re-infection rates involve sampling stool and/or urine, usually 12 months after treatment, which therefore occurs just before the scheduled annual re-treatment, which has given time for re-infections. So, again, we have the uncertainty as to the contribution of inadequate parasite clearance or that existing parasites were cleared and there has been transmission or re-infection.

Worms in Disguise

One of the most fascinating aspects of schistosome research relates to how the larvae of all schistosome worms manage to survive unharmed when they invade the human body and make their way to the liver where they then develop into adults. Having paired up male and female, how they then survive within the human host's body, apparently undetected, is a mystery. They survive for an estimated minimum of about six years, with longevity having been recorded over 20 years in exceptional cases. Understanding the mechanisms by which these worms manage to effectively hide within the body might provide valuable information which can be transferred to improve the survival rates from organ transplants.

Much of the core material which informs immunological theory today has been derived from studies of schistosomiasis and leishmaniasis (another parasitic disease caused by a protozoan parasite which is transmitted by sandfly bites), looking at how they bypass our immune system. For example, the Th1/Th2 hypothesis, which relates to the differing roles of various T-helper cells (core cell types in the human immune system) was developed and demonstrated through studying worms.

Researchers from the University of Georgia in the USA, who are part of the wider schistosomiasis research community, suggest schistosomes rely on a combination of mechanisms to achieve this 'disguise'.

The human host does produce a range of immune responses to the invading worms but for some reason they are not powerful enough to kill them. Several possible explanations exist.

Firstly, the worms have the ability to adopt some of the host antigens and thus masquerade as host tissue. (When lecturing about this aspect of the schistosome life cycle I refer to the schistosomule using a 'Harry Potter Invisibility Cloak'.)

Secondly, and perhaps a more complex suggestion, worms may modulate the host immune response to stimulate regulatory cells influential in down-regulating other immune responses capable of harming the worm.

Thirdly, it is possible that schistosomes have a high turnover of surface membrane molecules so that when host immune effector cells attach to the schistosome surface, they slough them off with their outer membrane.

Finally, the critical worm antigens which could stimulate human immune responses are hidden within the adult worms and are only exposed when the worm is broken open by the action of praziquantel.

Despite these various hypotheses, the available evidence is insufficient to establish one of them as dominant, and with the arrival of new tools which allow for genetic manipulation, there are likely to be more possible theories around the corner. (I prefer the Harry Potter hypothesis.)

Making Praziquantel Taste Better

There seems to be little enthusiasm among scientists and pharma to find an alternative drug to praziquantel, but as stated earlier a consortium spearheaded by Merck is working to develop a less bitter paediatric formulation of praziquantel which will be suitable for treating infants aged from 6 months to 5 years.

This initiative has reached phase III testing of their product in Cote D'Ivoire and Kenya, and the product should be on the market before too long (maybe 2022). Another improvement being developed is the synthesis of the isomer of praziquantel, which apparently is not only effective but also tasteless. The L rotamer[1] is believed to be this isomer and if this is proven the product will provide the answer to improving the taste and effectiveness of the schistosomiasis treatment.

Gates Foundation and the SCORE Programme – Creative Thinking for Schistosomiasis Control

Professor Dan Colley of the Center for Tropical and Emerging Global Diseases (CTEGD) at the University of Georgia (UGA) was asked by the Gates Foundation in 2008 to set up a programme to engage people from a range of countries, organizations and backgrounds for a common cause – to improve the implementation of schistosomiasis control. This was because of a paper he wrote in 2007 defining all the research questions in the schistosomiasis world to which there were as yet no answers! (Colley and Secor, 2007).

And so Dan became the Director of the Schistosomiasis Consortium for Operational Research and Evaluation (SCORE), based at UGA, bringing together scientists from immunology, malacology, social science, epidemiology, mathematical modelling and population genetics, to name just a few. They provide the Gates Foundation with research sub-plots on which to focus so as to speed progress in the control and elimination of the disease. The team visited each of their country field programmes regularly in Kenya, Tanzania, Cote D'Ivoire, Niger and Mozambique. The various projects collected a massive body of data, which has now been published and sums up Dan's career achievement.

Dan is another scientist who has contributed so much to the progress in the control of schistosomiasis, bringing together research and implementation communities. There are some people that one interacts with over and over again, and gains a great respect for (which I hope is mutual). Dan is one of these people because, like me, he has devoted his career to achieving the vision of fighting diseases of poverty globally, but especially schistosomiasis. He strongly supported the growth of research in the USA, initially as director of a laboratory at Vanderbilt University in 1971, then as Director of the Parasitic Diseases Branch at the CDC before moving to be head of CTEGD. Internationally, his collaboration in the early days of his career was in Brazil, but then included scientists who rose to hold senior positions at the Kenya Medical Research Institute. In between, he fulfilled a ten-year

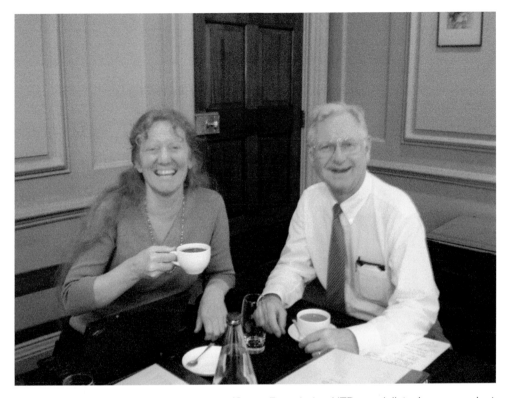

Fig. 17.2. Dan Colley and Julie Jacobsen (Gates Foundation NTD specialist who as a project officer to SCI was *ex officio* on the SCI advisory board – see Ch. 7).

collaboration in Egypt. From 1988 to 1998, he was on the panel supporting the project I led in Egypt (SRP) and he visited me there at least once a year, working with Egyptian researchers in the Nile Delta on the immunology of schistosomiasis.

SCORE protocols

One of the major components within SCORE was entitled 'Gaining and sustaining control'. Standard protocols were developed by 2011 for implementing in their selected countries and the plan was to test several chemotherapy strategies in four different endemic settings, namely: high *S. haematobium*, low *S. haematobium*, high *S. mansoni* and low *S. mansoni*. The purpose of this project, which finished in 2020, was to look at these four different endemic settings and implement four different strategies for control:

- comparing annual school-based treatments versus community-based treatment; and

- testing the effectiveness of annual treatments versus reducing treatments by taking 'praziquantel holidays' in alternate years.

The project plans required many technicians in each country examining very large numbers of stool and urine samples, and quality control was most important to ensure the results were meaningful. The results of the SCORE programme were not conclusive but the programme achieved many publications which were brought together in a 2020 edition of the *Journal of the American Society of Tropical Medicine and Hygiene* (Colley *et al.*, 2020).

Note

[1] Praziquantel is a mixture of optical isomers. Only one is effective (R) and the other (S) causes the bitter taste.

18 Recognition for SCI Work

Over the period 2003–2019, the achievements of SCI were widely recognized: by Imperial College, by the Committee awarding the Queen's Anniversary Prize (2007); by the Royal Society of Tropical Medicine and Hygiene (2004 and 2015); by the presidents of Burkina Faso and Niger (2006); by the University of St George's (The Mike Fisher Prize 2014); by the American Society of Tropical Medicine and Hygiene (2012) and with award of the Dominique Kyelem Prize (2018).

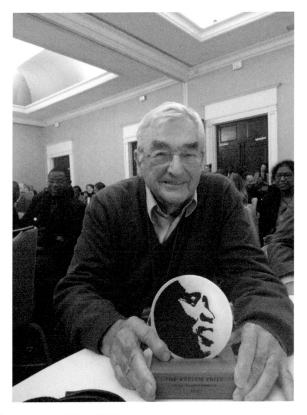

Fig. 18.1. Dominique Kyelem Prize 2018.

© Fenwick, Norris and McCall 2022. *A Tale of a Man, a Worm and a Snail: The Schistosomiasis Control Initiative* (A. Fenwick *et al.*) DOI: 10.1079/9781786392558.0018

The Queen's Anniversary Prize 2007 to SCI and Imperial College

Every two years, all the postgraduate institutions in the UK (there are 620) are invited by the Royal Anniversary Trust (directed by Peter Chenery) to submit one entry for the Queen's Anniversary Prize. In 2006, Professor Leswek Borysiewic suggested to Sir Richard Sykes, the Rector of Imperial College, that I prepare an application on behalf of Imperial College as the 2007 (Round 7) entry, describing SCI and what the project was doing for the health of millions of African children. My staff and I spent many a long hour preparing a careful manuscript to submit to the trust, but we received a lot of help from the trust secretariat and the college during the preparation. After the submission there was a long wait while all the entries were assessed. I had almost forgotten about the entry when Sir Richard Sykes telephoned me personally with the news that our submission had been successful and we were one of the 20 Queen's Anniversary Prize medal-winners for 2007.

As a winner I was invited to a dinner at the Guildhall in February 2008, attended by the Queen and the Duke of Edinburgh, on the evening before the actual presentation ceremony at Buckingham Palace. I was allowed to bring seven guests to the Guildhall to form a table of eight dignitaries, and then to Buckingham Palace where we would be ten people, five staff from Imperial College plus five students. In addition to the Imperial professors, I invited Alan McCormick (Chairman of the Board) and Mark Lorenson (CEO) from Legatum to thank them for their recent support to SCI. On the next day I was joined at the palace by the Rector of Imperial College, Sir Richard Sykes, Professor Steven Smith (who by then had taken Borys' position as Dean of the Faculty of Medicine at Imperial College), Sir Roy Anderson, Head of Department of Infectious Disease Epidemiology (DIDE), and Professor Joanne Webster (DIDE).

The five SCI staff members who joined us were Dr Lynsey Blair, Dr Fiona Fleming, Dr Mike French, Dr Artemis Koukounari and Dr Elisa Bosque-Oliva. Sir Richard and I were presented with the medal and the scroll by the Queen and the Duke, and then our team of ten was greeted informally by the Queen and the Duke in the gallery at the palace, with the other 19 winners and their teams. It was a very exciting day for us all.

But there was more recognition to come from the Anniversary Trust. Some years later, Peter Chenery contacted me to say that the Queen had commissioned him to write a book on this Anniversary Prize to celebrate 20 years of its award and that he had selected SCI and Imperial College to be one of the ten prizewinners highlighted. Then he added that a short film was to be made of three selected projects from the 200 winners, and SCI was one he wanted to include. A recognized documentary film-maker named Louis Poltnoi was chosen to make the films but when he came to SCI at St Mary's he expected to make the film there. I explained that our work was mainly in Africa, but he said he had no budget to travel there. If the film was to reflect SCI's work it had to include footage from Africa and so SCI agreed to pay for him and his cameraman to fly to Uganda, and he filmed some

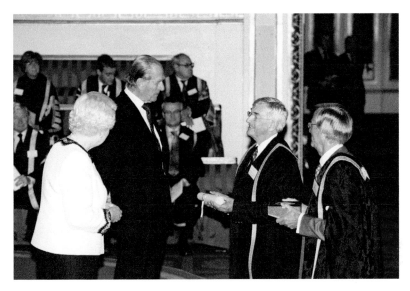

Fig. 18.2. Buckingham Palace, 2008; Alan receives the Queen's Anniversary Prize with Sir Richard Sykes.

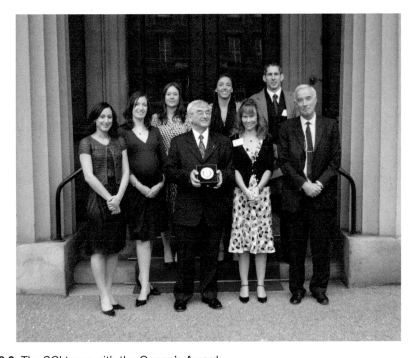

Fig. 18.3. The SCI team with the Queen's Award.

footage there with Dr Narcis Kabatereine in a starring role. We were very thrilled with the result, which can still be seen on the Queen's Anniversary Prizes website (http://bit.ly/31GRm0e) and indeed on Youtube (http://bit. ly/3mk1unk).

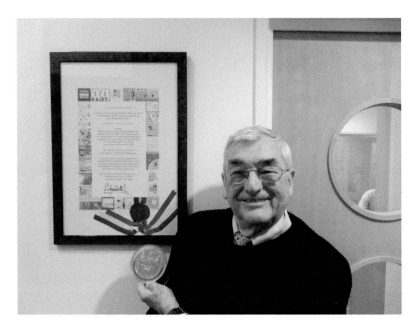

Fig. 18.4. Queen's Anniversary Certificate and Medal being shown by Alan.

The Mike Fisher Award 2014 (and a teaching position at St George's and Northumbria University)

Indirectly, George Nelson was responsible, posthumously, for me receiving the Mike Fisher award from the University of St George's on the Caribbean Island of Grenada. Mike Fisher was one of the team that developed ivermectin for Merck in the 1980s. He retired to Grenada and taught at the university until his death. The Mike Fisher Award was set up in his memory and was awarded annually to contributors to the control of NTDs. Cal Macpherson was the parasitologist at St George's in 2010 but 40 years earlier, he and I were both working in East Africa in the 1970s under George's supervision. However, although we knew of each other's existence, we never managed to meet because I was in Tanzania and he was in a remote spot (Turkana) in Kenya. Cal ended up, and is still, on the staff of the Medical School of St George's, and when George was ill, around 2008, we somehow managed to make contact with each other and meet up when he visited the UK. Cal needed someone to teach a cohort of his students who were spending a year in the UK at Northumbria University in Newcastle and asked if I would mind filling the void. I agreed, and, as a result, ended up working with Professor David Holmes in Newcastle and lecturing there on NTDs. I have done this every year since, even lecturing virtually on a Zoom call in 2021.

In 2014, at the House of Lords, I was presented with the Mike Fisher Award for my life's work by Baroness Howell (who is from Grenada). I was very honoured to receive this accolade and have joined some very special people who have received this award since its inception in 2004.

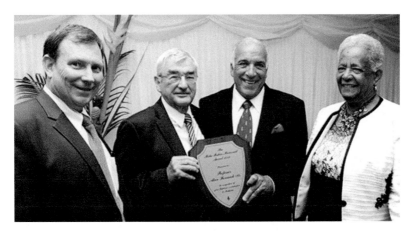

Fig. 18.5. The Mike Fisher Award received by Alan Fenwick.

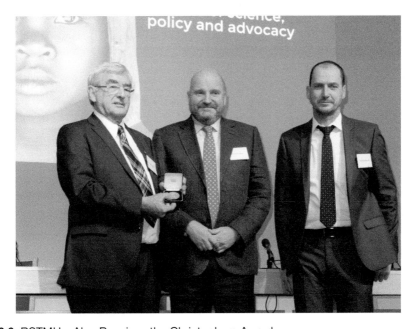

Fig. 18.6. RSTMH – Alan Receives the Christophers Award.

The Sir Rickard Christophers Medal 2015 (RSTMH)

Having successfully nominated Dr Andrew Davis for this medal in 2003, it was a great thrill to be nominated in 2015 by Professor Russell Stothard and to be awarded the medal at the RSTMH annual meeting, with the citation being read by Simon Bush from Sightsavers. This medal, too, is a reward for a lifetime of achievement and is only awarded every three years, which makes it a very special honour and made me very proud.

Box 18.1. Press Release for Knighthood from Burkina Faso 2007 – Schistosomiasis and STH and LF Integrated!

Members of Schistosomiasis Control Initiative receive the "Chevalier of the Ordre National" from Hon. Alain Yoda in Burkina Faso

By Laura Gallagher
21 June 2007

The contribution of Imperial's Schistosomiasis Control Initiative (SCI) to the health of people in Burkina Faso was recognised by the country's Ministry of Health on 12 April 2007.

The Honourable Alain Yoda, the Minister of Health of Burkina Faso, presented members of the SCI team with the "Chevalier of the Ordre National" at a ceremony in Tenkodogu, in the presence of the Governor of the Province and over 2,000 dignitaries and guests.

The SCI, which is directed by Professor Alan Fenwick, from the Division of Epidemiology, Public Health & Primary Care, aims to assist countries in sub-Saharan Africa to control the parasitic disease schistosomiasis and STH infections. It was set up in 2002 with a £20 million grant from the Gates Foundation.

Mr Yoda presented the Chevalier medal and ribbon to Professor Alan Fenwick, Mr Howard Thompson, Dr Albis Gabrielli, Dr Bertrand Sellin and Mme Elisabeth Sellin. The awards recognise the assistance given by the SCI in implementing the schistosomiasis and STH control programme, and the way in which the SCI has encouraged the establishment of integrated control of Neglected Tropical Diseases at a national level.

At the ceremony, Professor Fenwick thanked the Minister for the honour bestowed upon the SCI team, and paid tribute to the dedication and hard work of the Burkina Faso team, which is led by Dr Seydou Touré. Professor Fenwick also thanked the Gates Foundation for their contributions to the SCI and to the Burkina Faso Programme.

On winning the award, Professor Fenwick said: "This award shows that the Government of Burkina Faso appreciates the efforts of SCI in improving the health of the Burkinabe, and the fact that treatment against schistosomiasis, STH and lymphatic filariasis has now been scaled up to cover the whole country."

"Three challenges remain for the next three to five years: first, to continue the existing coverage with annual treatments; second, to scale up treatment of trachoma; and third, to integrate the treatments into a package of treatment. This will hopefully be achieved with funding from the United States Agency for International Development, through their NTD programme," he added.

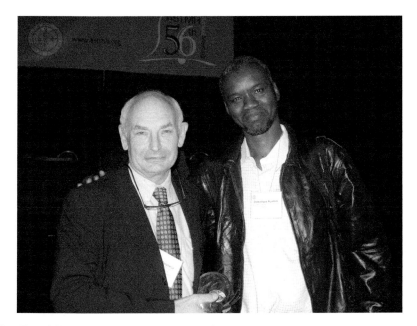

Fig. 18.7. David Molyneux with Dominique Kyelem.

Dominique Kyelem Medal 2018

In 2017, the third annual award was awarded, jointly, to Dr Mwele Malecela from Tanzania and Professor David Molyneux from Liverpool because the committee vote could not separate these two most worthy scientists.

Mwele had been instrumental in establishing a countrywide campaign against lymphatic filariasis, and such is her expertise and experience that she is now (in 2019) responsible for NTDs in WHO Geneva. I was honoured to receive the fourth prize, awarded in 2018, and in 2019 Dr Johnny Gyapong was the prizewinner for his work in Ghana and his international expertise on committees for WHO, again for the NTD control campaigns.

Chevalier Awards from Burkino Faso and Niger

I have already spoken of the 'Chevalier experience' in Burkina Faso, and, as I say in the press release (Box 18.1): 'This award shows that the Government of Burkina Faso appreciates the efforts of SCI in improving the health of the Burkinabe, and the fact that treatment against schistosomiasis, STH and lymphatic filariasis has now been scaled up to cover the whole country.'

It was indeed recognition for the entire SCI team back in London and in Burkina Faso. We received similar recognition in Niger. By 2006, the SCI team had visited Niger several times, and formed a working relationship with RISEAL a French-based NGO headed by Dr Bertrand Sellin and his wife Elizabeth. The Ministry of Health, particularly the Director of Health

Services Dr Ali Djibo, had embraced the programme right from the outset, when it must all have seemed rather a wild possibility. Dr Ali immediately recommended the then minister to sign up, and both that minister and his successor supported us fully. Their mobilization efforts, greatly aided by the RISEAL Director Dr Amadou Garba's efficiency, produced a very effective programme under the most difficult conditions.

Through RISEAL Burkina Faso, whose local director was Dr Seydou Touré, SCI donated significant assistance to the Ministry of Health in the form of support for a RISEAL office, transportation (a motor vehicle and 17 motorcycles to help district health workers), plus praziquantel and albendazole for the annual treatment of people living in endemic areas of Burkina Faso.

In heavily infected areas, all the residents were offered treatment, and in areas where the prevalence was lower, school-age children were targeted. The Niger government appreciated the efforts that SCI and RISEAL had made for the health of school-age children in particular and invited us to accept a Chevalier de L'Ordre Nationale, a Niger-specific, gold-medal

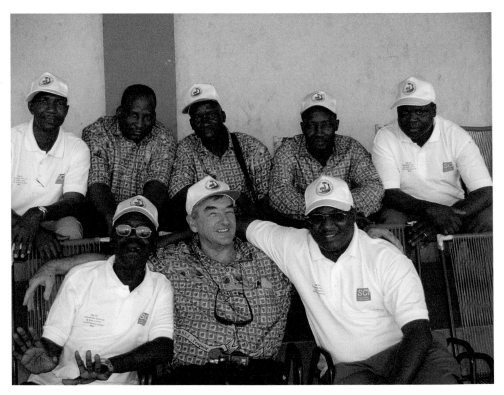

Fig. 18.8. The West Africa team wearing the shirts associated with the launch of the Burkina Faso programme and for which we received the Chevalier award. (Front row, left to right) Ali Landoure (Mali), Alan Fenwick, Amadou Garba (Niger); (back row, left to right) Adama Keita (Mali), Seydou Touré (Burkina Faso), unidentified (Mali), Robert Dembelé (Mali) and Moussa Ouedraogo (Burkina Faso).

equivalent to a knighthood. In addition to myself, Howard Thompson (the Deputy Director of SCI and a French speaker), Dr Albis Gabrielli, our Programme Manager for Niger, and Dr Bertrand Sellin (President of RISEAL, France) were also invited and we were thrilled to be presented with our medal and a certificate of appreciation by the Minister of Health. The award of this medal to foreigners was a significant honour for which we all are very grateful.

19 Accelerating Control of NTDs and Schistosomiasis in Particular, 2008–2020

Public healthcare in sub-Saharan Africa, even post-COVID-19, has reached a critical mass that promises positive change for almost one billion of the world's poorest people. This change has been driven by an expansion of interest in the ironically termed 'neglected tropical diseases' or NTDs, and the success of integrated control programmes for them. Now, elimination by 2030 of most NTDs is in sight because of the continued support by public–private partnerships of pharmaceutical company drug donations, bilateral donors (UK and USA), fundraising organizations (GiveWell, GWWC, The END Fund), implementing NGOs (RTI, SCI, GAELF) and the ministries of education and health in the endemic countries. Much remains to be done to bring about elimination, but the word 'neglected' in the context of tropical diseases may not hold true for much longer.

NTDs have gone from being virtually unknown in the 20th century outside the poor and rural areas of the world, to a situation where in the early part of the 21st century over one billion treatments are being delivered each year.

A Little History of NTD Control Successes

As mentioned previously, the control of NTDs had started small with the support of Bill Gates in 2000, but the successes achieved in the early years of the initiatives he funded in Africa had seldom been told until 2012. Frankly, this was because only the rural poor suffered these diseases and they mostly suffered in silence. Worms like hookworm had been largely eradicated from wealthier Europe and North America.

The year 2008 was a turning point with a string of official announcements and pledges aimed at combating NTDs, and this was followed by key events in 2012.

2008 USA and UK give millions for NTDs

First was the wonderful news that the US government had pledged $100 million for research and control into NTDs for a five-year programme. A few months later, the British government pledged £50 million, also for five years.

The stated goal of the US-Bush initiative was to reduce and eventually control the seven major NTDs (lymphatic filariasis (LF), schistosomiasis, trachoma, onchocerciasis, and three soil-transmitted helminthiases (STH)) by integrating treatment programmes for more than 300 million people in Africa, Asia and Latin America. The British government took a different approach and funded three specialist groups to each implement control against the diseases in which they specialized. So SCI was funded to control schistosomiasis and STH in selected countries, GAELF was funded to control LF, and APOC was funded to control onchocerciasis.

In addition to simply funding treatment programmes for these diseases, the UK grant included support for more healthcare workers and provision of water filters and safe water supplies. These would ensure people in countries affected by NTDs had access to clean water and learnt how to avoid exposure to water-borne diseases.

My colleagues and I had calculated in 2006 that an investment of $1 billion over five years would provide a combined treatment package for nearly everyone in sub-Saharan Africa, bringing the major NTDs under control. Suddenly, with the US and UK awards, we were one third of the way there.

Not all the NTDs are confined to Africa, however, and so we were aware that more funds would be needed for the control of the parasitic diseases outside of Africa (in particular LF and STH).

It is worth mentioning that $1 billion over five years was a minute amount in comparison to funds then already awarded by the US government for research and control of both HIV (in PEPFAR) and malaria through the President's Malaria Initiative (PMI). But $1 billion was substantial in comparison to the minimal amounts available for treating the NTDs in 1999, before the Millennium Development Goals (MDGs).

Zamalek, an Egyptian doctor uses the gents, and A&E at Watford

A nasty accident in 2008 but a happy ending

I attended a conference in Liverpool organized by David Molyneux, and on the way home I left the train at Watford Junction and tried to phone the taxi driver I had booked. Unfortunately, I was going downstairs at the time and took a terrible fall. I knew it was bad – but not how bad. Several people kindly came to my assistance thinking I had simply twisted an ankle but I just said: 'Please, I cannot stand, I need an ambulance'. An ambulance duly arrived and took me to Watford General where I was deposited in my wheelchair clutching my laptop and a small suitcase of overnight clothes. I was out of sight of the A&E desk, and in a corner opposite the gents toilet. I might have sat there a long time but after an hour of inactivity I was saved by a doctor (he had a stethoscope round his neck) who came out of the toilet; I called 'Excuse me'. I explained my predicament and said I was a Professor at Imperial College. 'Oh,' he said, 'I trained there' (which was a good first step). He asked my name and I asked his. He said his was difficult because he was Egyptian, and I pronounced his name with my obvious Egyptian accent and he was impressed. 'You speak Arabic,' he said, and I replied, 'Aiwa lakin Shwoya' (yes, some). He asked where I had learned it and I said Cairo, where I had lived and worked for 14 years. He asked me where I had lived. I replied 'Zamalek'.

'Where in Zamalek?'

'Hassan Asim Street.'

'Oh, what number?'

'Number 6.'

'Amazing,' he said, 'I and my family live in Number 4!'

So, within 20 minutes I had X-rays done and a consultant to see me. It transpired that I had snapped my tendon and needed surgery, and I was four months in plaster and on crutches. But I made a good recovery and even made some new friends who walked our dog Simba every Saturday and Sunday morning until I recovered (thanks, Pat and Chris).

There was a plus side to the post-operative care. I travelled to the USA during the last part of my recovery, wearing a knee brace and walking on crutches. This meant I was taken through customs and immigration both at Heathrow and Dulles airports in Washington, DC, in a wheelchair. I have never before, or since, cleared those airports, both in and out, so quickly. Now I am back to the time-honoured method of joining the queue.

Tropical disease advocates call on G8 for finance in 2008

David Molyneux, myself and Peter Hotez called on the Group of Eight (G8) nations to establish a global financing mechanism to ensure a more sustained global financial commitment to fight NTDs. By 2015 we were still trying to expand the support for MDA against NTDs to make full use of the fantastic leverage opportunities related to pharmaceutical company donations. I think it's fair to say that they all listened sympathetically to our arguments but did not pay much more than lip service when they said they supported our programmes. As time went by, the British and American aid programmes continued to support mass treatments against NTDs but the other G8 countries did not offer major support.

Gates moves funding from treatment to operational research

In a move that was a great disappointment to me and the SCI team, the Gates Foundation decided not to renew their support for SCI and our expansion into more countries in Africa. Their argument, as I understood it, was that we had completed our proof of principle and it was up to other donors to support further treatment. Instead, they changed tack from implementation and funded operational research to improve implementation of schistosomiasis control (see Chapter 17, SCORE, Partnerships). In November 2008 they announced an award of US$34 million to set up SCORE at Georgia University in Athens, USA, headed by Professor Dan Colley.

The Elders focus on NTD cause

Finally, the Elders, a group formed under the inspiration of Peter Gabriel, Richard Branson and the late Nelson Mandela, convened with the Secretary General of the UN, Ban Ki-moon and adopted the NTD cause. The group included leaders from UN agencies, foundations, the private sector and civil society who all pledged to highlight the plight of the world's poorest inhabitants and discuss strategies to combat NTDs.

WHO DG Chan pushes NTDs up the agenda

The WHO Director General, Margaret Chan, throughout her time in office, from the time of the London Declaration in 2012 until 2019, went to great lengths to publicize the need for concerted action against NTDs in a number of speeches she made on the international stage including the World Health Assembly in 2013 (Box 19.1).

The progress towards elimination of NTDs became her star achievement in many people's eyes. All of the above drove the increasing visibility of NTDs within the international news agenda and, in turn, this generated further political responses.

Box 19.1. World Health Assembly resolutions 2013.

WHA 65.21 urges member states to proceed towards elimination of schistosomiasis.
WHA 66 12. 2013: The following actions are essential for maintaining the progress already made and further reducing the global impact of neglected tropical diseases:

a. To prioritize prevention, control, elimination and eradication of neglected tropical diseases in national health, political and development agendas.
b. To sustain the development and updating of evidence-based norms, standards, policies, guidelines and strategies for prevention, control and elimination of neglected tropical diseases.
c. To collect additional information on the costing of interventions and of the socioeconomic impact of neglected tropical diseases.
d. To collaborate with partners in areas such as resource mobilization and programmatic management in order to implement interventions to prevent and control neglected tropical diseases.
e. To ensure predictable, long-term financing for sustained interventions against neglected tropical diseases.
f. To build national capacity to implement preventive chemotherapy interventions, expand those interventions nationwide and maintain a national coverage of at least 75% of the populations in need, for as long as necessary to reach the targets in the WHO's roadmap for work to overcome the global impact of lymphatic filariasis, onchocerciasis, schistosomiasis, soil-transmitted helminthiases, and blinding trachoma.

During Chan's time, a dedicated WHO NTD department was formed with Dr Lorenzo Savioli as director until 2014, followed by Dr Dirk Engels, then Dr Gautam Biswas and, in 2019, a longer-term leader, Dr Mwele Malacela from Tanzania.

Rolling Out Integrated MDA for NTDs in Earnest in 2008

A toolbox to integrate NTD programmes

As you may have realized, most efforts to control and eliminate the NTDs have been achieved through individual global health partnerships aiming for either elimination or the lesser target of morbidity control using prevention chemo-therapy (PC). Of 92 public–private partnerships (PPPs) listed against specific health problems around the world, six key ones are aimed at specific NTDs and work within sub-Saharan Africa. These organizations function in parallel using a toolkit of one or two drugs deployed over large areas and populations. Together, four drugs form the backbone of NTD treatment: albendazole, iver-mectin (Mectizan), praziquantel, and azithromycin (Zithromax).

In 2012, more than 100 million Africans in around 30 countries were targeted to receive free treatment. This was a huge achievement, but such was the expansion of the NTD control efforts that by 2016 the outreach target figure was 1 billion – and one billion treatments were delivered!

The individual NGOs and the NTDs they treat can be found listed in Table 19.1.

Table 19.1. PPPs engaged in vertical programmes for neglected tropical disease control in Africa. (From Molyneux *et al.*, 2005.)

Programme	Disease target	Major drug(s) Used
Schistosomiasis Control Initiative	Schistosomiasis and STH infections	Praziquantel and albendazole
Partnership for Parasite Control	STH infections	Albendazole and mebendazole
Human Hookworm Vaccine Initiative	Hookworm	Albendazole and Vaccine Development
International Trachoma Initiative	Trachoma	Azithromycin
Global Alliance to Eliminate Lymphatic Filariasis	Lymphatic filariasis	Ivermectin and albendazole
African Programme for Onchocerciasis Control	Onchocerciasis	Ivermectin
Drugs for Neglected Disease Initiative	Focus on trypanosomiasis and leishmaniasis	Drug development
WHO Programme to Eliminate Sleeping Sickness	Sleeping sickness	Suramin and melarsoprol

DOI: 10.1371/journal.pmed.002033G.t002

Rapid Impact Package promoted by GNNTDC

The GNNTDC accomplished and oversaw massive progress in fundraising and knowledge promotion, and its closure in 2015 was an indication of its success. One of its key activities, key to the success of the integrated programmes, was the promotion of the Rapid Impact Package, the combination toolkit described in Chapter 15.

Zanzibar

One of the first countries to integrate their NTD control activities was the island of Zanzibar, where the schistosomiasis and STH control activities were conducted in conjunction with an LF programme. This resulted in the ministry of health giving an annual dose of ivermectin with albendazole, and a twice-yearly dose of praziquantel with albendazole.

It makes such sense to integrate these MDA programmes in order to jointly increase efficiency and coverage of vulnerable populations and optimize cost-effectiveness due to economy of scale. Integrating the various NTD partnerships across Africa proved a formidable task, but by 2008 NTD programmes were all grouped collectively at the WHO headquarters in Geneva and at the regional directors offices (in Africa, Harare and Brazzaville). Most ministries of health in Africa followed this lead and consolidated their NTD programmes under one director.

Operational Challenges of Integrated Control of NTDs

Above and beyond drug donations, a major challenge for integrated programmes lies in the complexity associated with accurately mapping disease distribution, the mobilization of resources and the delivery of drugs at the right time and to the right populations. How this is handled is detailed below.

Mapping at the micro level

Mapping on a micro level – at the village or district level – is conducted to determine geographical overlap between different diseases. To do this we developed rapid and inexpensive assessment techniques such as screening for uro-genital schistosomiasis via school-based questionnaires. Mapping of LF in all endemic countries has used a simple but accurate antigen detection assay. Using funding from the Queen's Jubilee Trust, all trachoma-endemic districts were mapped in a massive global project (Global Trachoma Mapping Project) run by Sightsavers.[1]

Overlapping spatial data

After mapping individual NTD distributions, it is necessary to overlap spatial data to determine areas of co-endemicity. Using a combination of geographical information systems, remote sensing techniques and spatial statistics, implementation plans can be made. Usually, one district health officer may already be responsible for implementation of all the control programmes but may now need to better co-ordinate and streamline activities.

Logistics

Given that most drugs are donated, the costs implicit in NTD programmes relate to treatment-associated activities. These would include the cost of training and advocacy, transport of drugs and people, and *per diems* for staff while away from their homes. Integrating NTD programmes aimed at millions of people demand expert planning at both a strategic and tactical level. A large dose of good logistics is required. Drugs need to arrive in the country in plenty of time and be transported to communities on the correct days and in the correct quantities. Sometimes, certain equipment will be necessary; health education needs to be arranged and delivered prior to treatment; training needs to be provided, and monitoring and evaluation carried out. Failure to deliver on any of these requirements could derail a programme (remember Tanzania – see Chapter 3).

Safety: co-administration of drugs

Having planned and co-ordinated the MDA programmes, consideration needs to be given to the safety of co-administering drugs. For example, when the LF control programme was proposed, before combination therapy between albendazole and ivermectin or diethycarbamazine was given, surveillance of adverse effects due to the combinations was conducted through pilot studies. The WHO has recommendations on combination use; for example, it approves administration of praziquantel with albendazole and with ivermectin. However, surveillance of adverse effects is still likely to be conducted before wide-scale use of this three-drug combination. Use of azithromycin in addition to those three drugs definitely requires further surveillance and administration and so treatments are split into two MDAs per annum.

Monitoring disease prevalence

Another challenge inherent in integrated programme delivery is how to monitor and evaluate (M&E) disease prevalence, intensity and morbidity.

When only single treatments were delivered, each control programme used its own M&E process and could attempt to evaluate the positive effect of the drug regime they delivered. In an integrated delivery programme, only the combined effect of the integrated programmes can be measured – M&E would then produce an overall measure of health, well-being and equity but no indication of the contribution of each individual drug. The development of how best to implement M&E of integrated NTD programmes was attempted by SCI after they delivered integrated treatments to the residents in Uganda and Niger. The results were difficult to interpret, and since 2015, SCI has reverted to assisting the ministries of health to deliver all the drugs needed to control the NTDs prevalent in any one area. M&E has reverted to measuring separately the reduction in prevalence and intensity of just schistosomiasis and STH.

Many of the other cross-over challenges related to combined programmes such as training, social mobilization and community-based distribution mechanisms should, in principle, lead to considerable cost savings, providing further evidence to support the oft-cited fact that integrated NTD programmes are the best buy in healthcare today.

Benefits of Integrated NTD Programmes

Combining experience

Poverty is the common denominator which underlies all the NTDs, and co-ordinated mapping of each disease highlighted the high degree of geographic overlap and co-endemicity between the seven most prevalent NTDs. However, the efficient use of available funds is dependent on the strategy and infrastructure in place to utilize them, and the separate NTD organizations provided a diversity of valuable experience to each other to develop integrated programmes. For example, APOC had expertise in reaching some of the remotest and most vulnerable populations through its extensive network of community drug distributors. Using their experience, the distribution of the additional drugs (praziquantel and azithromycin) and reaching the target populations of the different NTD organizations were integrated into the APOC model.

Double benefits – other diseases also respond to NTD drugs

The integrated treatment programmes brought additional, unplanned but very welcome, benefits. The drugs we delivered, coincidentally treated even more neglected conditions than those directly targeted. For example, people with food-borne trematode infections and skin infections such as scabies and lice were beneficiaries of praziquantel and ivermectin, respectively. Also, over time, it was realized that the widespread use of azithromycin against trachoma had improved the health of children because the treatment had impacted other childhood bacterial infections, including some severe ones caused by group A streptococci but also ear infections, diarrhoea, yaws and the sexually-transmitted diseases such as chlamydia and gonorrhoea.

The Rapid Impact Package can treat some symptoms without us knowing which infection had caused them. The best example is anaemia, which can be caused by schistosomiasis, hookworm or trichuriasis, but was reduced in the communities by the package. Reduction in anaemia improved appetite, activity and school performance in children and reduced their susceptibility to other infections. A particular benefit of reducing anemia was to pregnant women because anaemia is associated with maternal morbidity and a low birthweight in babies. Thus, our integrated NTD programmes improved child health, maternal health and birth outcomes.

Value-for-money healthcare

By any standards, the costs associated with integrated NTD programmes for large populations are incredibly good value and bring to the poorest people in the world an immediate improvement in health and quality of life. For a modest US$0.40–0.50/person/annum, the integrated control of NTDs – with annual delivery of donated drugs – alleviates a host of debilitating symptoms, minimizes further infection and improves the long-term prospects in education and earning potential for millions of people.

In 2005, our calculations suggested that if we could raise US$200 million each year for five years, over 500 million individuals (representing the majority of the population of sub-Saharan Africa) could benefit from preventative drug treatment. This action would rapidly contribute to poverty reduction and take steps toward achieving seven of the eight Millennium Development Goals (Fenwick *et al.*, 2005). In 2015, aiming to achieve the SDGs, the WHO estimated that there was a need to target up to 1.4 billion people for coverage, requiring an investment of an estimated US$2.8 billion in the period 2015–2020 (WHO, 2015).

Recognizing that delivering donated medicines to over a billion people is a complex undertaking, Fitzpatrick *et al.* (2016) ran a literature review on costing studies for six NTDs and developed web-based software that can help to monitor value for money. It calculates the 'specific unit costs against which programme budgets and expenditures or results-based pay-outs can be benchmarked' (Fitzpatrick *et al.*, 2016).

For schistosomiasis and STH, the bang for the buck in 2021 is still estimated to be less than 50 cents/person/year, and that is based on donated praziquantel and albendazole. The money is spent on staff training and local personnel costs plus travel and transportation of drugs. All these costs have been published by Fiona Fleming of SCI.

NTD drug delivery does not need medical personnel

Another key factor instrumental to the success of NTD programmes is that medical personnel are not essential to attend MDA sessions, other than in a supervisory capacity. As with SCI-assisted programmes, the key to success has always been careful planning with local teams, the mobilization of local community health officers and teachers, and engagement of school-children through health education. Health education reassures children, clarifying the reasons for drug treatment and encourages compliance. It is because the drugs are so safe that specially trained doctors and nurses are unnecessary – one or two days of training for community leaders is usually sufficient, providing the infrastructure to deliver medications is already in place.

In the case of schistosomiasis, our training first explains about the taste of the tablet and the need for food to be taken beforehand. It then prepares the staff for possible side-effects, highlighting vomiting, stomach-ache and headache. Describing the life-cycle promotes longer-term behavioural changes to reduce water contact where possible and to improve hygiene. That particular message is needed to complement and eventually change disease-related activities. However, behavioural changes can take many years. Having lived in sub-Saharan Africa for over 34 years, I regularly point out that when temperatures reach the high 80s and early 90s, it is difficult to tell a child not to cool off in a local lake or river.

Impact of NTDs on malaria and HIV

Advocates of NTD programmes think beyond just treating NTD infections and strongly believe that there are gains for malaria and HIV control through combating NTDs. Studies suggest around 90% of helminth-infected individuals are at risk of co-infection with malaria (Brooker et al., 2006). Other research highlights the immunosuppressive features of helminths, especially the STHs, schistosomes and filariae, and their possible role in increasing susceptibility to HIV/AIDS, TB and malaria (Babu and Nutman, 2016; Druilhe et al., 2005; Fincham et al., 2003). Chronic infection with helminths may impact the immune responses to some vaccines such as for TB (Cadmus et al., 2020; Maizels and McSorley, 2016; Zakeri et al., 2018) and for tetanus.

A significant component of the morbidity associated with malaria results from the severe anaemia so often seen in children and pregnant women. This effect is amplified by the blood loss and iron-deficiency anaemia of hookworm and schistosomiasis. It has also been suggested that schistosomiasis and hookworm might weaken the immune system predisposing an individual to more severe malarial attacks.

Thus, co-infection with malaria and NTDs adds up to a potentially very damaging combination where malaria patients are worse off if co-infected with NTDs than if they have malaria alone.

The Early Integrated Programmes

The ultimate proof of integration is, of course, seeing how the fundraising and roll-out of programmes translate into lives saved and disease
burden reduced on the ground. Integrated NTD programmes were
quickly established in most countries across sub-Saharan Africa and ministries of health combined their separate NTD programmes into an 'NTD
department'.

The first examples, after Zanzibar, included Burkina Faso where
schistosomiasis and STH treatment programmes have now been integrated
with LF and onchocerciasis programmes since 2008. In Niger, 8.4 million
people (62.7% of the country population) were treated in the integrated
MDA during April 2008 and this has continued. In Uganda, the combined
NTD programme initially targeted 9 million people treating them for
onchocerciasis, LF, schistosomiasis and STH, but expanded into trachoma
after mapping for that disease was completed (Hotez *et al.*, 2006) (Fig. 19.1).
Funding for this came from the Global Fund, PEPFAR, the President's
Malaria Initiative and DFID.

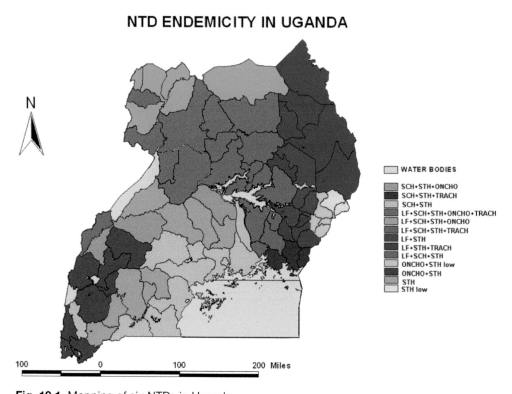

Fig. 19.1. Mapping of six NTDs in Uganda.

COVID-19 – Impact on Current Integrated Programmes

Scaling up preventive chemotherapy for NTDs presents opportunities not just for integrated delivery, but also for integrating mapping, monitoring and post-intervention surveillance as programmes reach the elimination phase (Baker *et al.*, 2010). Experience of integrating NTD control using rapid impact packages for more than one disease in Uganda, Tanzania, South Sudan and Mozambique, informed a detailed 'how to do it' article by colleagues Narcis Kabatereine, Mwele Malecela, Sam Zaramba and others (Kabatereine *et al.*, 2010). This article emphasized, as this book has done, that much hinges on forging partnerships with ministries and international agencies, down to village level. At this point, in 2010, disease mapping was done separately for each disease but overlap was then established.

In 2021, there is now successful experience of integrated disease surveys – where several diseases are mapped by the same team at the same time. This approach is seen as the 'logical tool' to achieve the 2021–2030 road map targets for NTDs. They need careful planning, and training of field workers takes longer as they need to learn about several diseases. But the advantages include that one sample can provide data for several diseases (e.g. sero-surveys), a reduction in implementation costs for remote communities and the chance to use a standardized survey process with a single platform for electronic data capture and management (along the lines of the Global Trachoma Mapping Project/Tropical Data systems[1]) (Harding-Esch *et al.*, 2021).

All this good news stands to be undermined or at least held back in the current pandemic and post-COVID era. The economic impact of COVID has increased the number of people living in extreme poverty from 650 million in 2019 to an estimated 766 million in 2020 (Hotez *et al.*, 2021). According to these authors, Nigeria, DRC and India in 2017 were the three most endemic countries for NTDs and are currently being hit the hardest in terms of COVID–associated poverty. Their fear is that economic derailment through COVID in these countries, and in others such as Yemen, Burkina Faso, Tanzania (with long-standing successful integrated control programmes), will slow global efforts to eliminate NTDs. COVID-19 is testing the health systems and economies of all countries: there is a risk that donors may cut funding to NTD programmes and health staff in Africa will be diverted. WHO guidelines and MDA activities were suspended for a period in 2020, providing an opportunity for transmission of infection to increase. Drug supply, either through expiry of drugs during the suspension of programmes or from reduced manufacturing, together with limited delivery, are very real issues.

On the other hand, NTD programmes, if supported, can offer resources to fight COVID-19 whilst delivering on their original agenda, namely smartphone technology for COVID-19 surveillance, an existing network of community drug distributors and scaling up of WASH messaging. Hand, face and limb hygiene are key components of NTD interventions for LF, STH and trachoma (Molyneux *et al.*, 2020).

Note

[1] Global Trachoma Mapping Project, led by Sightsavers, ran from 2012 to 2016 and mapped 29 countries using smartphones to collect data from 2.6 million people. Its work carries on as Tropical Data, which so far has surveyed 6 million people in 40 countries.

20 The Last Mile

With the meteoric rise in annual treatments since 2012 now bringing us close to ending NTDs as public health problems in many countries, we could be said to be in the 'last mile', reaching for their final elimination. For me, the last mile includes the transition for SCI to new management and their leaving the umbrella of Imperial College. I handed over the reins of SCI as a 'benign dictator' to the senior management team of four amazing colleagues, who led SCI initially within Imperial College and then moved out of Imperial in 2019 to become a standalone charity, The SCI Foundation.

This chapter provides the 'state of play' on NTDs in various countries in 2019 and describes the reasons behind SCI's bid for freedom.

SCI Becomes an Independent Charity 2019

During my last two years at SCI, at Wendy Harrison's request and in anticipation of my retirement, we brought in a consultant team to review our management structure, our procedures and our position within Imperial College. My position as Director had been helped massively by being a professor in this prestigious academic institution, but when I retired, the new Director would probably not be appointed a professor there, and meanwhile we were all very aware of some constraints on SCI within Imperial.

What is your charity number?

The first major, long-term constraint was not the fault of the college. Although the SCI brand had become well known, globally, the first thing that potential donors asked was almost always, 'What is your charity number because we cannot find you?', and we would have to explain that we did not have charity status in our own right but that we were covered by the charity status of Imperial College. This was not always easily accepted and I am sure that some donors were put off by this unusual situation. Charity status is important to donors, especially those based in the USA, as it brings tax advantages to the donor.

© Fenwick, Norris and McCall 2022. *A Tale of a Man, a Worm and a Snail: The Schistosomiasis Control Initiative* (A. Fenwick *et al.*)
DOI: 10.1079/9781786392558.0020

A second constraint was that while our position in the college was as a prestigious programme bringing in many millions of pounds in donations and bringing better health to millions of people, we were no longer the strong research organization publishing many scientific papers that we had been in the early days of SCI, when our work was ground-breaking.

Once we had proved that our disease-control strategies were successful, SCI had become more about implementation than about high-profile academic and operational research. Imperial College is very well known for its purely academic research, which meant that our position within the college, perhaps, raised eyebrows at the senior levels.

Bureaucracy delays drug deliveries

Finally, there was the constraint of increased bureaucracy. The college was forced into a higher level of accountability because of some scandals in the education sector. For international reasons, transferring money into and out of the college now had to cope with stringent financial restrictions and the fear of money laundering.

A major issue was that the legal agreements that needed to be negotiated between the college and recipient countries had become tedious. Previously, I could visit countries and sign contracts with ministers of health; now SCI senior staff could no longer sign agreements, everything having to go through the college lawyers in the Joint Research Office (JRO). The JRO was apparently seriously understaffed to deal with all the contracts that came across their desks and ours were particularly complicated. Finalizing them was so time-consuming that our ability to work in the countries in a timely fashion, and therefore our schedule of drug deliveries, was being delayed. By 2013, the situation had become untenable to the extent that SCI ended up employing a lawyer to sit in the JRO.

With these constraints becoming more difficult to navigate, soon after my handover the new senior management team made the decision, with the agreement of the SCI advisory board, to leave the comfort of Imperial College and apply for its own charitable status. The process was never going to be easy but, finally, in mid-2019 the SCI Foundation received its own charity number (1182166), rented new premises in south London, and both the team and the money donated to SCI moved away from Imperial College to a new registered charity home.

New procedures, new management team

The review of our processes and the development of our new management structure were overseen by staff from Accenture Development Partnerships (ADP), which, as part of its corporate responsibility, offers services to the development sector at non-commercial rates. As a result of their recommendations, our procedures were improved, our staffing plan was amended to reflect different skills and responsibilities, and our programme management was strengthened. The most important change was a strengthening of our financial department and the recruitment of a qualified accountant to head up the sub-unit. I and the senior SCI team members were very grateful to ADP for their input and the new SCI management team were thus prepared and ready to launch out as an independent charity.

I am sure the split from Imperial College was not easy to organize but both parties agreed that it was the best way forward for SCI – once I had left – to continue their efforts to raise extra funding, apply for grants and compete for contracts.

The Schistosomiasis Control Initiative Foundation

The new independent structure would be better able to assist more endemic countries in a more streamlined way, and so this has proved to be. When I left in December 2016, the new management team comprised Dr Wendy Harrison as Director of SCI, Dr Lynsey Blair as Head of Implementation, Dr Fiona Fleming as Head of Monitoring, Evaluation and Research, and Ms Najwa Abdallah as Chief Financial Officer. This team has ensured the transition was smooth and I am thrilled to recount that it has been a great success.

In 2019, the SCI Foundation (SCIF) became a charity, with premises in Edinburgh House, 170 Kennington Kane, London SE11 5DP (charity no. 1182166). Because SCIF has this charity number, its position in society and in

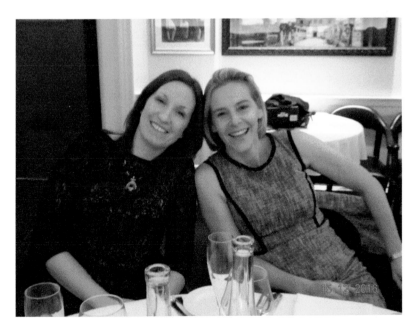

Fig. 20.1. Dr Lynsey Blair, Head of Implementation, and Dr Wendy Harrison, Director of the SCI Foundation.

the charity world is much clearer to supporters and donors than when SCI was under the umbrella of Imperial College. Being independent brings greater flexibility in terms of recruitment, pay and conditions. SCIF will, in future, be fully transparent and in control of financial resources and risk systems specially designed for a charity working in Africa. The main supporters of SCI have congratulated Dr Harrison and her team for making this bold step to stand alone, and have pledged to continue their support to the de-worming and schistosomiasis control work of the organization.

Where are we today?

When I retired in December 2016, some 18 countries had been reached by the SCI and over 200 million treatments had been delivered with SCI assistance. Every country in Africa has now been mapped for distribution of a number of 'neglected tropical diseases'. Every country has started a schistosomiasis treatment and control programme, with around 85 million people in Africa receiving free treatment in 2018 alone. School health programmes to treat parasitic worms have been established across Africa.

According to WHO, in 2021, preventative chemotherapy is now required in only 52 endemic countries with moderate to high transmission. Another 26 have low transmission and so do not require preventative chemotherapy (see Fig. 2.1).

I wonder if Bill and Melinda Gates realize just how much the population in Africa have to thank them for their improvement in health and quality of life – but also how much more could have been done more quickly if they had not finished supporting SCI so early in our existence.

Since leaving Imperial, SCIF has continued to support over 40 million treatments every year and maintains its cost-effectiveness by treating three children for every £1 sterling donated. For the tenth consecutive year, SCI, and now SCIF, has been named as one of the top charities by GiveWell (www.givewell.org).

SCIF's first annual report in November 2020 stated that, in 2019, it reached 48 million people with a total of 61.5 million treatments, and highlighted their contribution to the new three-year DFID programme ASCEND. The programme is a consortium (Sightsavers, Mott MacDonald, Liverpool School of Tropical Medicine and SCI Foundation) whose target is to work towards elimination of the five NTDs in West African countries. SCI Foundation is leading efforts in Cote D'Ivoire, Liberia and Niger. In East Africa, another ASCEND project is underway fronted by Crown Agents and my colleague Narcis Kabatereine is involved again in continuing his mission to eliminate schistosomiasis in Uganda.

During the difficult period 2019/20, due to a restriction of activities because of COVID-19, SCIF still managed an impressive set of achievements under the ASCEND umbrella treating 1,782,425 in Cote D'Ivoire, delivering 5,599,611 treatments against LF, onchocerciasis, schistosomiasis and STH in Liberia, and supported training of almost 80,000 community drug distributors, 7205 health workers and 5314 teachers in the ASCEND countries in West Africa.

Table 20.1. WHO recognizes 20 NTDs.

Buruli ulcer	Mycetoma and mycoses
Chagas disease	**Onchocerciasis (river blindness)**
Dengue and chikungunya	Rabies
Dracunculiasis (Guinea worm)	Scabies and other ectoparasites
Echinococcus	**Schistosomiasis**
Food-borne trematodes	**Soil-transmitted helminths**
Human African trypanosomiasis	Snakebite envenoming
Leishmaniasis	Taenia and cysticercosis
Leprosy	**Trachoma**
Lymphatic filariasis (LF)	Yaws (Treponema)

State of Play with NTDs by 2019

NTD control programmes are fortunate in that safe and effective drugs exist and are made available to the rural poor because they are donated by drug companies and donor agencies. These drugs reduce NTD infection rates to levels that, until relatively recently, were a pipe dream. There are now 20 NTDs recognized by the WHO.

Table 20.1 shows these diseases, with the five controlled by preventive chemotherapy in bold type. In 2016, WHO launched ESPEN (Expanded Special Project for Elimination of Neglected Tropical Diseases), a five-year programme to provide technical and fundraising support for elimination of the five.

Guinea worm: eradication is near but has a setback

Guinea worm is the nearest to eradication, and in 2015 we were all poised to celebrate eradication with the prevalence having moved from 21 countries in the late 1980s, when there were some 3.5 million new cases each year, to just 22 cases worldwide in 2015. Sadly, in 2020, eradication seems to be impossible because of some new data. In 2016, there were 25 new cases, globally; in 2017, 30 cases; in 2018, 28 cases; and in 2019, 48 human cases reported.

The change has been due to the discovery of an animal reservoir, mainly in dogs (over 1000 infected in Chad) but also in some cats and baboons (the latter in Ethiopia). The final disappointment was when two cases were discovered in Angola, which was previously thought to be free of guinea worm. On the positive side, no human cases were found in 2019 in the previously infected countries of Mali, South Sudan and Ethiopia. Eradication campaigns in Chad now include burial of fish guts, treatment of surface water and containment of infections in dogs as well as people, in order to reduce the animal reservoir.

Lymphatic filariasis (in Africa, Asia and the Americas)

Progress has been made towards elimination with some countries having reached, or are approaching, elimination and therefore have qualified for cessation of MDA. Togo has been the first country in Africa to be declared free of LF, and MDA has stopped in Cameroon and Malawi. Two states in Nigeria (Plateau and Nasarawa) are also free from LF as a result of the Carter Center program there.

However, in 2019, an estimated 341 million people still required annual MDA in Africa of which over 211 million did receive treatment in 2018, and in virtually all countries in Africa, MDA is well underway. In South-east Asia, over 523 million people qualify for MDA and over 335 million received treatment with ivermectin plus DEC plus albendazole. Most of these (almost 261 million) were in India, but Indonesia, Myanmar, Nepal and Timor sites were also treated. In the Western Pacific region, coverage was good in the Philippines and Fiji, but still areas of Papua New Guinea require better coverage.

In the Americas, LF has been all but eliminated by frequent MDA although sites in Guyana and Haiti still need to reach elimination and stop MDA.

As for morbidity, due to LF, almost one million cases of lymphedema were reported in South-east Asia and almost 100,000 in Africa. In men, the number of hydroceles[1] reported was 452,891 in South-east Asia and 109,771 in Africa.

Onchocerciasis

With river blindness virtually eliminated, and APOC closed, the required progress to the elimination of the parasite onchocerciasis and the stopping of annual ivermectin treatments continues, led by ESPEN under the auspices of WHO.

The major triumph in 2017 was the cessation of treatment for the first time in six foci in Ethiopia, although there were still 191 districts to continue. Plateau and Nasarawa states in Nigeria stopped treatment in 2018, again thanks to the detailed support of the Carter Center. The Mectizan Donation Program (MDP), supported by Merck in the USA, has committed to continue their donations to both the onchocerciasis-infected countries but also to countries where Mectizan is given in conjunction with albendazole against LF.

In 2018, WHO reported that although some 149 million people were treated, an estimated 217 million individuals still qualified for treatment in 23 countries and so the Mectizan donation was being fully utilized. All but 25,000 of those needing treatment were in Africa, with the remainder in just a few small foci in Central and South America.

In 2019, over 153 million people received treatment. Twenty-five thousand were in Central and South America, and 721,000 in eastern Mediterranean

regions. Of the 218 million people, globally, who required preventive chemotherapy, 70.4% were reached.

The move to elimination is well underway. More than 1.8 million people
(in Equatorial Guinea, Gabon and Guinea) now live in areas where transmission has been broken and thus no longer need MDA. Scale-up mapping for
elimination of the disease has been conducted in Chad, Congo, Côte d'Ivoire,
Democratic Republic of the Congo, Equatorial Guinea, Ethiopia, Kenya,
Mali, Nigeria, Senegal and Sudan.

Trachoma

After the donation by the Queen Elizabeth Jubilee Trust, most of the trachoma-
infected foci in the world have been mapped, and the global elimination of
trachoma is within reach. Based on data in 2019, some 142 million people live
in trachoma endemic areas in 44 countries.

Azithromycin (Zithromax), donated by Pfizer through its corporate
responsibility team, was used to treat over 89 million of these people in
preventive chemotherapy. The damage to eyes of over 146,000 individuals
was operated on in 2018. By 2019, Pfizer had donated over 500 million doses
of Zithromax and, in the 20 years since the donation programme started,
over 100 million people have received treatment. Since 2012, nine countries
have had elimination validated including Oman, Mexico, Iran, Morocco,
Ghana, and now, in 2021, Gambia. Another four are awaiting validation, but
for global elimination, additional input is needed to provide access to clean
water and sanitation.

Schistosomiasis and STH

The progress towards elimination of schistosomiasis and STH has been
slower than with the other preventative care diseases above, mainly because
the donation of praziquantel against schistosomiasis and both albendazole
and mebendazole against STH took longer to expand in scale than did the
donations against onchocerciasis, LF and trachoma.

However, the WHO December 2019 weekly epidemiology report highlighted that 76.2 million school-age children (SAC) and 19.1 million adults
received praziquantel during 2018. These numbers were 41.6% of those
deemed to need treatment but the SAC coverage was a very satisfactory
61.2%, while treatment of adults was lower. Despite these good results, some
countries had yet to submit their treatment figures. The countries to deliver
the most treatments were Nigeria (11.4 million), Burkina Faso (9.9 million),
DRC (7.8 million), Malawi (7.2 million), Tanzania (6.5 million) and Ethiopia
(6.4 million).

It is calculated that 38 million children received albendazole or mebendazole to treat STH concurrently with praziquantel. In non-schistosomiasis

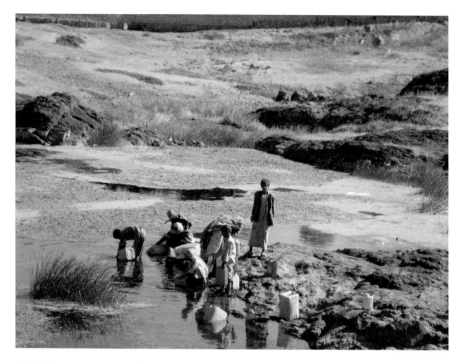

Fig. 20.2. Yemen – water collection is an opportunity for schistosomiasis transmission.

areas, many STH treatments were delivered – 120 million preschool children and 456.3 million SAC were treated with either albendazole or mebendazole.

Outside of the WHO Africa region, there are two countries in the eastern Mediterranean region of WHO (Sudan and Yemen) endemic for schistosomiasis and in need of MDA. In South-east Asia, only Indonesia needs treatment. In the Americas, Brazil was the only country to report treatments, while in the Western Pacific, Cambodia, Lao and Philippines reported treating some 0.6 million SAC.

E-Merck donates praziquantel against schistosomiasis and in 2016 donated the 500-millionth tablet. On average, 2.5 tablets are required to treat a child, and the company has provided 250 million tablets a year since 2017. It is also part of a consortium developing a paediatric formulation of praziquantel which will be less bitter and easier for preschool children to swallow. This formulation has now reached a phase III trial in Cote D'Ivoire and Kenya; and funding is in place, as of 2021, to identify the best approaches to achieve widespread acceptance and access to this treatment (ADOPT implementation research program – data from Global Schistosomiasis Alliance, 2021).

In 2014, E-Merck recognized the need for an umbrella organization to co-ordinate activities against schistosomiasis and employed Dr Lorenzo Savioli as director of the GSA when he retired from WHO. The GSA is a virtual secretariat and has grown in acceptance by the schistosomiasis community. In 2017, Dr Savioli moved on, and Professor David Rollinson became Director, and the base for GSA moved to the Natural History Museum in

London. David recruited Anouk Gouvras to support the secretariat as communications and programme manager, and I spent two years contributing to the promotion of the GSA and schistosomiasis control activities.

The New NTD Roadmap 2021–2030, and a New NTD Day

A special day in the progress towards control and elimination of neglected tropical diseases was 30 January 2012, with the meeting in London hosted by Bill Gates and the signing by many participants of the London Declaration. Also in 2012, the World Health Assembly passed a motion at their annual meeting in May calling for the adoption of a target – elimination of some NTDs by 2020.

This ambitious target proved, for many countries, unattainable, but a new target has now been set and in the (virtual) 74th World Health Assembly of 2021 a new NTD road map was agreed for the period 2021–2030. In addition, that special day was formally recognized by the WHA and adopted as World NTD Day, with all the activities and focus such days bring.

Informally celebrated by the NTD community in 2020, the second day in 2021 coincided with the launch of the NTD road map on 28 January. Events were held throughout the world but especially innovative was the illumination of several iconic buildings 'to shine a light on the suffering these diseases cause' (www.who.int/news/item/27-05-2021-world-health-assembly-adopts-decision-to-recognize-30-january-as-world-ntd-day).

This push to eliminate NTDs is a serious movement and Dr Mwele Malecela, Director, WHO Department of Control of Neglected Tropical Diseases, is on record as saying:

> World NTD Day is in appreciation of the work spearheaded by the United Arab Emirates along with other Member States and partners to inspire and incentivize communities to fight these debilitating diseases. I am confident this recognition will further motivate everyone to work across sectors to implement the new road map, which aims to free over a billion people from these diseases by 2030.

> Hopefully, the now formal NTD day will raise much-needed attention and visibility to these diseases of poverty, and the 2030 target for elimination in many countries will be achieved.

Note

[1] Hydroceles are scrotal swellings. In LF, they are caused by the parasite: they are disfiguring and can impact fertility, mobility, and even ability to earn a living.

21 What Next for Alan?

So finally, at the end of 2018, the time arrived for me to retire from all the scientific posts I was holding and allow myself some leisure time at the ripe old age of 77. Margie has continued to work as a psychotherapist and we still live in Chalfont St Giles. I was able to retire with my three daughters settled in their own homes with apparently secure jobs and each with a husband and two children. After her graduation as a medical doctor, Janet, the eldest, specialized as an anaesthetist while working in a hospital in Reading, and then, when she had graduated to the Royal College of Anaesthetists, she moved to Perth in Australia for some work experience, accompanied by Kevin and their two boys, before returning to the UK to become a consultant. She finally accepted a post at Birmingham Children's Hospital as a consultant paediatric anaesthetist. Meanwhile, her eldest son and my eldest grandson, Peter, graduated from Leeds University and is now a teacher of Physical Education. Matthew, Janet's younger son, is currently studying at Nottingham Trent University.

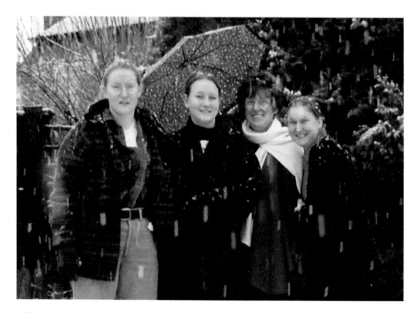

Fig. 21.1. Fenwick girls with Irene.

DOI: 10.1079/9781786392558.0021

Gill, meanwhile, having worked in TV production for a while, settled in Maidenhead about 35 minutes' drive from us, with husband Ben and two daughters. Ben is working in the music and film industry, while Gill works for the mobile phone company Three. Their two young daughters are very talented, with Izzy producing some amazing artwork and Georgie is really into gymnastics. They are both still at secondary school.

My youngest daughter, Helen, is in Liverpool working in a leisure centre, while husband Darren is a carer. Their daughter, Laura Jane, studies at a film school and son Brendan is still at school.

We enjoy family get-togethers on special birthdays and around Christmas time. These gatherings include my sister, who worked for the NHS in Liverpool for most of her life before retirement, and she lives in what was our family home in Liverpool. Of course, during 2020 and 2021, we have yet to get together because of the COVID pandemic, but as I get my second vaccination in March 2021, perhaps we will be able to get back to normal by the end of the year.

Life in Retirement: Teaching, the Rotary, Golf and Holidays in Africa

Meanwhile, I am leading a happy life in retirement. I have now stopped lecturing, and when the 2020 annual Global Health Course at Imperial College at the end of June was cancelled due to the COVID-19 pandemic, I decided to cancel all further courses. I am very active in our local Rotary Club where, in 2018 and 2019, we raised funds for Medical Detection Dogs. This charity trains dogs to fulfil a number of medical tasks including diagnosing people with diabetes as they approach a dangerous hypoglycemia; diagnosing prostate cancer and breast cancer at a very early stage; and even diagnosing malaria. Other dogs assist disabled people with their everyday life, for example acting as a hearing aid.

At home, Margie and I have our own dog, a yellow labrador named Lindi (already a star with Simba in another part of the book!), and she ensures I walk my 10,000 steps every day. These steps are added to at least twice a week by playing golf at a very hilly local course, Harewood Downs, near our home in Chalfont St Giles. In the home I now do most of the cooking and shopping, and some of the other household chores, but I have yet to graduate to hoovering and ironing to a satisfactory level of competence.

This enables Margie to continue her valuable work as a psychotherapist (payback for the many years of support she gave to me).

We have invested in a holiday home in Padstow to which we disappear for several weeks every year and let it out to visitors to that magical part of north Cornwall. We like to return to Africa once every two years, where we love visiting national parks in Kenya, Uganda, Tanzania, Botswana, Namibia and South Africa, watching game of all sizes and birds. However, after a wonderful visit to South Africa and Botswana in December 2019, we are wondering whether we will ever get there again.

Golf

On returning to the UK, I had promised myself I would continue with golf, but although I joined a local golf club (Harewood Downs) and vowed to play once a week, for 14 years I dedicated my time to SCI. Since I rarely played more than twice a month, I have never mastered the local conditions (especially playing in wind and rain) and over ten years my handicap crept up from a respectable 11 to 16 in 2016 and then up to 22 as it is today. I was convinced that one day I would reverse the trend, but since I retired and can now play three times a week, I find myself getting no better! I did have a purple patch and began to play closer to my new handicap, and in 2017, and again in 2019, I did manage to win two trophies – the Commodore Cup for over-70s and the Gregorian Cup for over-75s. Winning is something I will always enjoy, and at least we gained some very good friends in Terry and Chris Wood. Terry plays golf, and he and wife Chris have been a large part of our lives in Chalfont St Giles. I miss those regular golfing sessions so was very pleased when the COVID golf closure was over.

Rotary

In 2002, I did try to reconnect with Rotary, which had been a large part of my life in Egypt, and I joined the Jordans and District Rotary Club near our home in Buckinghamshire. I was quickly recruited to be the Chairman of the International Committee and my first task was to organize an overseas visit for the members and their wives. I selected Cairo, and a group of 14 (club members and wives) spent ten days based there. We visited El Alamein cemeteries from World War 2 on the Mediterranean coast, and all the sites in Cairo including the Zabaleen settlement on the Mokatim hills together with their church and old people's home. The final day we spent at the Giza pyramids and it was on that day that we had our only casualty to a bad stomach when one of our number was too ill to join us. Fortunately, he recovered well enough to fly home. After a couple of years at the club, my travel to Africa for SCI became so frequent that I took a leave of absence from Rotary but rejoined when I retired. I was voted in as President for the Rotary Year of 2019/20.

I was also thrilled that my friend Professor David Molyneux was awarded a CMG in 2020 for his lifelong dedication to NTDs, especially onchocerciasis and LF; and that Professor Peter Hotez, the most prolific writer of scientific papers I have ever known, still has time to follow me on Facebook and remains my very good friend despite being one of the most famous scientists in the USA (have you seen him on CNN where he has been regularly appearing as guest spokesperson on COVID-19?).

But Who Anticipated COVID-19?

While I would normally finish by saying 'long may this happy situation continue', events have overtaken these wishes, namely the pandemic caused by COVID-19.

Just three months before the first lockdown, Margie and I went to South Africa to visit with our old friends, the Donaldsons, and attend the wedding of their son Jason to his fiancé Meghan. We took the opportunity while there to drive the garden route from Cape Town to Port Elizabeth and then fly to Botswana to stay in a beautiful lodge in the Okavango Delta. How lucky we were to make that trip because who knows whether we will ever be allowed another overseas holiday.

Living in a bubble in Chalfont St Giles

For most of 2020, and now three months into 2021, I have lived in my 'bubble' with Margie, and we have hardly left our house, having human contact only once a day with dog walkers at a socially distanced 2 m apart. I leave the house every morning at 6.30 am, and we walk the same route every day through fields off Stylecroft Road. In those fields we met up with Lawrence Wolman and his golden retriever Bailey, and Chris Cole and her labrador Pippa, and her son's puppy, a small, active cavapoo called Indy.

That one hour was the total exposure to the outside world – no shopping, no golf, no weekly Rotary meetings, no restaurants, no visits to our holiday home in Padstow, and no tube into London to the College or to the theatre. My last five months (February–June 2020) as President of Jordans and District Rotary Club was a period of inactivity. We had to cancel our planned visit to the Medical Detection Dogs (MDD) – my nominated charity – to which we had donated £4500 and had a puppy named Jordans in gratitude. I had managed to visit their dog-training centre in Great Horwood, Buckinghamshire, just before the lockdown and saw dogs detecting cancer (breast, bladder and prostate), neurological diseases, bacteria and malaria. Since my visit, the MDD, in conjunction with the London School of Hygiene and Tropical Medicine, have trained dogs to detect COVID-19, and I expect to see sniffer dogs at airports before too long.

Golf and Rotary in lockdown

We had to cancel a golf competition for our Rotary members, a club visit to Norwich, and finally a club lunch at which I was to hand over the chain of office to Manjit Shihn. So that the handover could be seen by everyone, Manjit and I met in his garden while the rest of the club assembled in five different venues, each venue with six people in attendance (Rotarians and partners). I handed over the chain of office and this was observed by all via a Zoom link.

Where will it end? Will vaccination bring us back to normal? As I finish this book, the over 80-year-olds are being vaccinated and I have received two Pfizer vaccines 11 weeks apart with no side-effects.

Appendix: Honourable Mentions

Margie Wright – Born Wright and always wRight!

The Schistosomiasis Control Initiative owes much of its success to someone who is not on the payroll nor is recognized as having contributed to the scientific achievements of SCI. When I moved to the UK from Egypt to establish SCI at Imperial College with a frighteningly large grant from the Gates Foundation and no staff or equipped office space, I was hardly at home. Margie and I had bought a house in Chalfont St Giles because the purchase price was just affordable, yes, but mainly because of its location – less than 30 minutes by train to Marylebone Station, which is 12 minutes' walk to St Mary's Paddington, but it was also close to the M40, which would take us to our families in Birmingham, Liverpool and Dumfries.

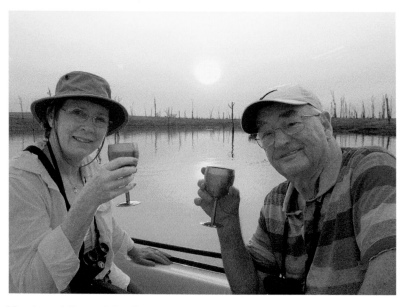

Fig. A1. Margie and Alan celebrating.

But guess who would unpack our belongings shipped in 20 boxes from Egypt? Who would buy all the furniture and other needs for the new house, set up bank accounts, credit cards, store cards etc., drive me to the station every morning for the 7 am train and pick me up in the evening? Margie was the answer, and I have to admit it took me some time to realize just how lucky I was, and am, to have her in my life.

Margie is not one to sit around, and so she continued her Samaritans work and then took a foundation course towards becoming a psychotherapist. Finding this an attractive potential occupation, she then embarked on a five-year course and became a fully qualified and accredited psychotherapist. Since her graduation, she has run a private practice and continued learning the subject of sensorimotor psychotherapy and the diagnosis and treatment of trauma. Meanwhile, she kept our house and garden in spectacular condition and bonded with my three daughters and their children in Solihull, Maidenhead and Liverpool.

Now that I have retired I have learned just how wonderful she has been to me while I travelled the world and received accolades, but I am pleased to say the boot is on the other foot now and in the world of psychotherapy it is she who is becoming widely recognized, and that makes me very proud.

Professor George Stanley Nelson (1923–2009)

Professor George Stanley Nelson loomed large in my life and career as you will have read. His qualifications fill two lines: MB ChB St And (1948) DTM&H Liverpool (1953) MD(1956) DAP&E(1960) DSc (1966) MRCP(1971) FRCP(1981) FRCPath.

When I knew him, George Nelson was Professor of Parasitology, first at the London School of Hygiene and Tropical Medicine (LSHTM) and then the Liverpool School of Tropical Medicine. He was born in Kendal, in the Lake District, and studied medicine at St Andrew's University and Dundee Royal Infirmary. After he qualified in 1948 he worked for two years in the UK until he left for Africa in 1950 to become a medical officer in the Ugandan Medical Service.

George's career and achievements in Uganda and Tanzania were amazing. As the doctor in charge of the West Nile District – an area of some 400,000 people – his specialist interest became parasitology and, in particular, leprosy, onchocerciasis, echinococcus and schistosomiasis, which were rife in that part of Africa. Whilst he was there, he studied for the Liverpool DTM&H and completed his MD. In 1956 he joined the Kenya Medical Service as a member of the Division of Vector Borne Diseases in Nairobi, which was a famous centre for research in parasitic diseases.

In 1959, while he was still in Nairobi, he passed the diploma in applied parasitology and entomology (DAP&E) at LSHTM. On leaving Kenya in 1963, he became, first, Reader in Medical Parasitology at LSHTM, and then, in 1966, he was appointed Professor of Parasitology and head of the department of helminthology. He spent 13 years in London and guided the department to become a major centre for studies in schistosomiasis, filariasis, onchocerciasis, hydatid disease and dracunculiasis. After London came the Liverpool School of Tropical Medicine in 1980, as Walter Myers Professor of Parasitology. Here he developed the units of immunology and genetics and promoted the hydatid research group in Turkana, Kenya, where there was the highest prevalence of the disease in the world.

George finished his career as President of the Royal Society of Tropical Medicine and Hygiene in the late 1980s. He wrote or contributed to over 180 papers on various aspects of parasitology but I knew him because in the West Nile area of Uganda, he carried out what was probably the most extensive survey of schistosomiasis ever undertaken, examining over 10,000 people. George claimed it was easy to obtain samples 'because all he had to do was get up in the morning, shoot a hippopotamus on the Nile and trade chunks of its meat for stool specimens'.

A stimulating and amusing lecturer he was constantly in touch with the areas of his research and concerned with the problems of underfunding in poor countries. It was typical of the man that having read my paper on baboons with schistosomiasis he followed up and became my mentor and friend.

Joe Cook – A Life-changing Acquaintance and Friend

When I first met Joe Cook he had joined the Edna McConnell Clark Foundation and visited me in Sudan. He came looking for projects to support for this foundation (founded with Avon Cosmetics funding), which, as part of their international support, had selected schistosomiasis as their tropical disease topic in which to invest their research portfolio.

Joe was thinking in terms of supporting researchers who were intent on developing a vaccine against schistosomiasis. He had spent some wonderful years in St Lucia as their chemotherapy doctor, and with his colleagues Pip Jordan, Mike Prentice, Bob Sturrock and others was the subject of jealous jokes because we in Africa all thought they had a cushy life in St Lucia where schistosomiasis was not really a serious problem, as it was in East and West Africa.

The St Lucia Schistosomiasis Project was funded by the Rockefeller Foundation out of concern for the spread of schistosomiasis in irrigation schemes, particularly in Africa, and chose St Lucia because it presented an opportunity to test different methods of control in quite separate valleys (chemotherapy, safe water and education, snail control or a combination of them). It ran from 1967 to 1981.

It was Joe (by now Director at ITI) who helped me get the Gates Foundation award in 2002 and it was he who suggested mediation when I wanted to base the SCI project in London and not with Michael Reich in Harvard, Boston.

What a Working Partnership and Friendship – David Molyneux, Peter Hotez and Eric Ottesen

Gary Weil, at a conference, showed a slide once which made me very proud – he took the picture of Mount Rushmore with four famous carved heads and replaced the presidential heads with those of myself, David Molyneux, Eric Ottesen and Peter Hotez and said these were the magnificent four people who had lifted NTD control to the place it is today. Of course, I know he could equally have added several more heads – Joe Cook (ITI), Adrian Hopkins (CBM and then MDP), Lorenzo Savioli and Dirk Engels (WHO), Roy Anderson (Oxford and Imperial College), Don Bundy (World Bank) and Uche Amazigo (APOC), to name but some. But that only made me more thrilled.

This is the place to perhaps mention a little more about Savioli and Otteson (since I have spoken about David and Peter in the last chapter of the book). Lorenzo Savioli started his work on schistosomiasis in Zanzibar and was there while I was in Sudan, but then he joined WHO in Geneva and built up an NTD department from nothing, and founded the Partnership for Parasite Control.

Today, that NTD department, from which Lorenzo retired in April 2014, is just booming with maybe 40 staff covering all the NTDs. How he achieved what he achieved we do not know, but he and his team were certainly effective, and Dirk Engels then carried on the good work until he too retired and the post went to Mwele Malecela.

The best advocate for NTD control for a decade, Eric Ottesen led the LF programmes from inside WHO at a critical time, and then went to Atlanta to continue his work. He eventually ended up with several jobs, including Principal Investigator for the Gates grant for operational research at the Task Force for Global Health, and Director of RTI's USAID-funded ENVISION project.

DFID Minister and Staff Supporting NTDs

I particularly want to mention some politicians (Lord Andrew Stone, Baroness Hayman, Sir Stephen O'Brien MP and Jeremy LeFroy MP) and DFID staff (Stewart Tyson and Delna Ghandhi).

UK Aid was channelled through the Department for International Development (DFID).

During the life of the SCI there have been a number of Secretaries of State for DFID, but the minister who was most influential for the development of aid to the NTDs was Sir Stephen Rothwell O'Brien, a British politician and diplomat. He was born in Tanzania on 1 April 1957 and educated in Mombasa, Kenya. He ensured that NTDs were included in the All-Party Parliamentary Group on Malaria (APPGM) and he was responsible for getting the first awards for work to combat NTDs through DFID.

Once the commitment had been made to support NTDs, it fell to the staff at DFID, Stewart Tyson and later Delna Ghandhi to implement the programmes and oversee the work of SCI and our partners at the Liverpool School of Tropical Medicine.

In 2015, much to the chagrin of the NTD community, Stephen was appointed as the United Nations Under Secretary General for Humanitarian Affairs and Emergency Relief Coordinator and was lost to our NTD cause. His place as Chair of the APPGM and NTDs was taken by Jeremy LeFroy, ably supported by Baroness Helene Hayman.

Another great supporter of SCI and NTDs who regularly spoke out in the House of Lords was Lord Andrew Stone, who served on the SCI advisory board from 2012 until 2017. I was fortunate to meet Lord Stone because I was sat next to him at a dinner in the Guildhall during the 2012 London Olympics, and we found we had a mutual interest in health matters. He invited me to the House of Lords to meet him and from that meeting we became friends and he agreed to support SCI on the advisory board.

The World Health Organization

I cannot stress enough the fantastic help I have had from, but also the pleasurable and productive interactions with, the WHO in general and with several individuals in particular.

From the top, the late Dr Lee and his successor Dr Margaret Chan both took NTDs from obscurity to where we are today, with Dr Tedros Adahanom continuing support through the new NTD road map for 2030. Dr Ian Smith and Dr Isabelle Nuttall in the DG's office regularly welcomed me in Geneva and listened to the advocacy which I and my colleagues bombarded them with. The NTD cluster was, during my time with SCI, under Assistant Director Generals, respectively, Dr David Heymann, Dr Endo and Dr Nakatani. It has been a pleasure knowing them all.

But the real colleagues have been the long-term friends Dr Lorenzo Savioli, Dr Dirk Engels, Dr Denis Daumerie, Dr Lester Chitsulo and all the other NTD staff. A special mention for Dr Albis Gabrielli who started his career as a programme manager for SCI before joining WHO. He has done so well and I am proud to have been there at the start of his rise to stardom (he hasn't yet quite risen as high as he will).

UNICEF and Others

Box A.1. Organizations that have supported SCI.

UNICEF kindly contributed de-worming drugs to support the programme in some countries in which SCI is operating.

Institut Pasteur, a French research organization aided monitoring and evaluation and collected data for the SCI in Mali and Niger.

The Wellcome Trust, the UK-based research funding charity, produced informative CDs[1] for SCI to distribute free upon request aimed at training medical workers in developing countries.

The Global Alliance to Eliminate Lymphatic Filariasis (GAELF) worked closely with SCI in several countries as we tried to integrate LF, schistosomiasis and STH control.

The **International Trachoma Initiative (ITI)** and the **African Programme for Onchocerciasis Control (APOC)** collaborated with SCI in planning integration of NTD programmes.

London School of Hygiene and Tropical Medicine (LSHTM) and particularly Simon Brooker for hosting Archie Clements as he developed his expertise on mapping disease in the early stages of the project.

The Centre for Neglected Tropical Diseases, based in Liverpool, moved from being a close ally to a full partner as DFID funding allowed us to work together to implement LF, schistosomiasis and STH treatment in eight countries after the 2010 award and even further when the next round of DFID funding was received. Liverpool led the implementation in Zambia and Mozambique.

Memorial to Dr Kyelem, Burkina Faso

Dr Dominique Kyelem had worked at various levels in various sectors of the health system of his country, Burkina Faso, for more than 14 years. During the late 1990s, he established the Burkina Faso National Programme for Lymphatic Filariasis, which he successfully led until 2007, and on which he based his PhD thesis. From 2007 until his untimely death, he was Programme Director for Neglected Tropical Diseases at the Task Force for Global Health in Decatur (Atlanta), Georgia, USA. Dominique had been a consultant for WHO since 2001 and had been supporting all the African countries to establish programmes towards the elimination of lymphatic filariasis. Dominique was admired and liked by his colleagues without exception.

A special memorial prize to commemorate the life and work of Dominique was established in 2015 by the Task Force and awarded in the first year to Dr Julie Jacobson, a most popular employee of the Bill and Melinda Gates Foundation, who had done so much to ensure funding for the NTDs.

In 2016, the prize was awarded posthumously to Vasanthapuram Kumaraswami, MD, PhD (1950–2016), a pioneer in the fight against neglected tropical diseases. The award was received by Dr Kumaraswami's children, Sameer and Manjusha Vasanthapuram, and recognized his lifelong commitment to bringing innovative solutions to the fight against NTDs.

In 2017, the third annual award was awarded jointly to Dr Mwele Malacela from Tanzania and Professor David Molyneux from Liverpool because the committee vote could not separate these two most worthy scientists. I was honoured to receive the fourth prize in 2018, and in 2019 Dr Johnny Gyapong was the prizewinner for his work in Ghana and his international expertise on the NTD control campaigns.

Individual Philanthropists

Giving What We Can, Good Ventures, MaxMind and Luke Ding

I would like to thank some specific philanthropists who, as individuals or as founders of organizations, made a huge difference to SCI. These are Toby Ord and Will MacAskill (Giving What We Can), Dustin Moskovitz and Cari Tuna (Good Ventures), Thomas Mather (MaxMind), Luke Ding and Mike Hauser.

GiveWell (www.givewell.org) evaluates charities, not just financially but also on how much good their programmes achieve per dollar spent.

Having organizations which evaluate charities in this manner may seem strange but the fact that they exist to support altruistically minded investors has made a huge difference to SCI and to other charities interested in improving the lives of those living in poverty.

Giving What We Can (www.givingwhatwecan.org) members take a pledge committing them to donate at least 10% of their income to relieve suffering caused by extreme poverty. As I write, they now have over 400 members who have, together, pledged $160 million.

When you read the annual grant-making by **Good Ventures** (www.goodventures.org) to SCI from 2011 to 2019, you cannot fail to be amazed at the support we received from them over the years. As of 2019, we had received a total of $23,750,000, which allowed SCI to reach out and help ministries of health in 16 countries to deliver some 50 million treatments against schistosomiasis and STH.

All this support has been on the recommendation of the GiveWell evaluators who, annually, look at SCI's expenditure over the previous year and the plans and budgets for the coming year, and then, based on these figures, make their recommendations.

Thomas Mather was another who contacted SCI (on behalf of **MaxMind**) via the GiveWell recommendation of SCI as a top cost-effective charity.

MaxMind, a provider of IP intelligence and online fraud detection tools, donates up to 60% of its corporate profits to good causes.

Luke Ding studied medicine at Oxford University, but subsequently switched to a career in finance. He came to us via Giving What We Can and donated an amount some 30 times larger than any other we had received at the time. This was on Just Giving and it arrived on my birthday. I immediately e-mailed him and invited him to visit SCI, which he did, and he then asked whether he could support a country. He decided for the first few years to continue the Legatum support to Burundi but later he wanted a new untreated country so that the treatments he supported would make a huge health difference. We listed all the available countries that met his criteria and he selected to cover Madagascar where the schistosomiasis prevalence was horrifically high. This became the successful Madagascar Schistosomiasis Control Programme.

It is difficult to express our appreciation of Luke's 'adoption' of SCI and the personal friendship which we enjoyed with him. Even after his direct financial support to SCI wound down, as he switched his financial direction, he remained close to SCI and Lord Stone and I enjoyed regular lunches with Luke for several years. After my retirement Luke continued his close association with SCI and was more than helpful when SCI moved from the Imperial College umbrella to become a free-standing charity, The SCI Foundation. It is no exaggeration to say the SCI would not be where it is today without Luke's support and millions of children have benefitted from regular treatments thanks to his direct financial contributions.

Legatum, Geneva Global and the END Fund

Together, these three organizations picked up the banner for the NTDs and raised funds to a level that was to dream of back in 2006 when the Gates money was likely to finish and the NTD programmes were in danger of running out of funds. I am proud to have been in at the beginning of Geneva Global's and Legatum's interest in NTDs and indeed at the launch of the END Fund in 2012. Their support to SCI over the years has been magnificent and I enjoyed working closely with the team. Today the END Fund has grown into a big player in the fight against NTDs, and I salute their team members with whom I have had the pleasure of working, including CEO Ellen Agler, plus Warren Lancaster, Elisa Baring, Kimberly Kamara and Karen Palacio. The team has now grown as fundraising has been so successful.

Mike Hauser, the racing vet comes into my life

Philanthropy is generosity in all its forms – 'time, talent and treasure' given to help make the lives of other people better. And Dr Mike Hauser gave generously of his time and expertise. Mike came into my life after he and his family were caught in Sri Lanka in the 2004 Boxing Day tsunami, which affected several countries. His family were caught by the massive waves and one of his daughters (Grace) was badly injured. He suffered some leg injury but his wife and other daughter (Ann) escaped relatively unscathed. Prior to the tsunami tragedy, Mike had been the senior veterinarian to the stars of the Godolphin Thoroughbred Racing Stables based in Dubai and Newmarket.

His life was totally changed by the tsunami and he took leave of absence from the stables. He moved to Geneva and while his daughters were in hospital there he decided to roam the world. His wanderings took him to Nepal. While trekking there he met farmers whose yaks were suffering a strange infection which Mike diagnosed as a worm causing neurocysticercosis. The cure for this parasite was the drug praziquantel. He googled praziquantel and my name came up as the most prolific user of praziquantel and so he visited me at SCI in London. I agreed to help him with a small supply of praziquantel which he then took with him back to Nepal and gave it to the farmers. Mike and I became friends, and he became fascinated with schistosomiasis and offered to help SCI in any way he could in the field or as a fundraiser.

I asked him to help us with a strange report from northern Ethiopia of a deadly liver infection in remote villages: an investigation by the Centre for Disease Control in Atlanta, USA, surmised it could have been caused by schistosomiasis. He went there with Anouk Gouvras who was then a PhD student in our department. They looked at the infected people, carried out stool examinations and searched for the host snails, and excluded schistosomiasis as a cause of the deaths. However, we wanted to find out the cause of what seemed to be a very deadly epidemic (the initial outbreak in Tigray 2001 led to 591 cases by 2009). Because the disease affected the liver we consulted Professor Mark Thursz, a liver specialist surgeon at Imperial College, and he took over the research with his student Oliver Robinson.

The disease was finally identified and named Hirmi Valley Disease. Mark and Oliver published their findings and the clinical presentation. In further investigations, significantly high levels of the alkaloid acetyl lycopsamine was detected in urine samples in 45 cases compared to 43 controls ($p=0.02$). It turned out that this novel disease was probably caused by co-exposure to acetyl lycopsamine and DDT, caused by storage of grain mixed with DDT and plants containing acetyl lycopsamine.

Mike helped me plan a treatment campaign against schistosomiasis in Ethiopia and represented SCI at various meetings at WHO in Geneva and in Uganda. In the end, in about 2014, Mike had placed his daughters in universities and so he decided to return to working as a racehorse vet, not in Dubai or the UK but in the USA. His premature death following orthopedic surgery was a great loss.

The three wise men of schistosomiasis – Andrew Davis, Pip Jordan and Gerry Webbe

To finish, let me acknowledge three other mentors and friends one generation ahead of me. I guess that every scientific discipline, and indeed every organization, has its share of characters, and the schistosomiasis world in the 1960s and 1970s was no exception. When I went to Tanzania as a 'new boy' to the schisto' world, I quickly learned about the famous three. They were Dr Rik Davis, Dr Peter (Pip) Jordan and Dr Gerry Webbe. There were others in the schisto' world, of course: Ray Foster, Fergus McCullough, Norman Crossland, Bob Sturrock and Joe Cook, to name some, but they will forgive me for remembering with fondness the three mentioned. In Sudan and in Egypt, these three stars were advisors to all my projects and regularly visited in the field.

Rik, when I first met him in 1966, was at the Malaria Unit in Tanga, Tanzania, which was, like TPRI, part of the East African Community. He then became an Assistant Director General at the World Health Organization, where he certainly made his name with the support WHO gave to the Phase III evaluation and then launch of praziquantel in the 1970s and 1980s.

Whenever they visited we had fabulous times, a critical but exciting evaluation of the work that we had achieved, followed by wonderful evening sessions with hot music provided by Rik at the piano and Gerry on drums. Gerry had contributed a lot to epidemiology research at the Schistosomiasis Unit in Mwanza, Tanzania, then ran a unit at Winches Farm near St Albans, an out-station of the London School of Hygiene and Tropical Medicine. His last triumph was the promotion of the molluscicide niclosamide developed by Bayer. Pip was the director of that same unit in Mwanza, and then he established and directed the St Lucia Project, which I have described elsewhere.

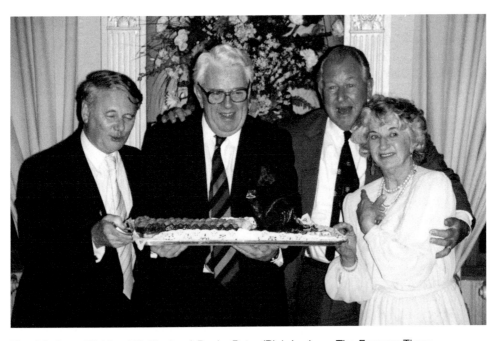

Fig. A2. Gerry Webbe, Rik (Andrew) Davis, Peter (Pip) Jordan – The Famous Three.

The West's Lopsided View of Africa

Since the millennium, the plight of Africa has generated an increasingly polarized response from different individuals and indeed different political groups. At one extreme there has been an impatient swell of Africa-fatigue in Western society where newspapers regularly write of the obscene wealth of certain African rulers, their lifestyles and their presumed corruption. Not only the leaders, though, because in some countries this corruption has spread downwards to most levels of society. Thus, many members of the general public believe that all African societies are corrupt and that the aid that is generously awarded by western governments does not achieve the good work for which it is intended.

At the opposite end of the spectrum we have governments and many celebrities (Bob Geldof, Bono and Richard Curtis to name a few), and, of course, the many organizations and philanthropists I mentioned earlier, who have embraced the cause of Africa, as well as millions of the caring general public. They have realized that in the poor rural areas of Africa so much can be done so easily to improve the health and quality of life of so many people who are suffering through no fault of their own.

Since 1990, high-profile events and networks such as Live Aid, the G8 initiatives, the Millennium Development Goals (MDGs), Tony Blair's 2005 Commission for Africa and, more recently, the Sustainable Development Goals (SDGs) have focused worldwide attention on helping sub-Saharan Africa drag itself out of the tragedy of extreme poverty which blights the lives of many of its 770 million inhabitants.

On balance, however, there is, sadly, an overriding public perception of Africa as a bottomless pit into which money is thrown and little benefit is gained. Only a minority of people living in the developed world fully appreciate that the underlying cause of any apparent lack of 'drive' in Africa may be poverty and ill-health related. Having lived in three countries in Africa for a total of 36 years, I firmly believed that parasitic diseases were (and still are) a major underlying constraint to the health and well-being of almost all rural Africans. With this conviction, I and like-minded colleagues wanted to rid the continent of these parasites.

We surely cannot help noticing that today, in Europe, most children tower above their parents – and I believe that the reason for their taller and fitter physique is due to the lack of any infection with parasitic worms during their early childhood, and the better hygiene and nutrition that the children of today have enjoyed.

We are advocating a change in global health on such a vast and fundamental scale that it will take years if not decades to achieve. However, we have already witnessed significant changes in the health of the people of Europe, and in parts of Asia – so why not in Africa? There are positive signs – since 1995 there have been increasing pockets of activity and local governance and community spirit achieving a change in circumstances, reducing poverty and improving health. For example, Uganda and its notable handling of the AIDs epidemic in the early 90s is a case in point.

One feature in common with nearly all notable success stories in Africa tends to be a determined effort to place the centre of gravity for any aid project within the local communities themselves, providing a strong sense of ownership and responsibility which, in turn, creates sustainability. For every single Western medical researcher there are millions of Africans who may benefit from their interventions; however, the engine to drive change, in terms of numbers and local knowledge, lies within the African people themselves.

Researchers, donors and policy-makers succeed when they embrace this concept and more than likely fail when they do not. In 1966, when I first went to Tanzania, local experts and Tanzanian university graduates were few and far between and most of the qualified researchers in the institutions in East Africa were expatriates from the UK. Fifty years later, many more of the African population are infinitely better educated but also healthier and more energetic to make change happen. The number of expatriates is now fewer in the scientific research institutes in East Africa, for example, as the local qualified scientists have filled the expatriate's shoes.

Gradually, the West is seeing that the 'undeveloped nations' such as Africa, a land of unique sights and sounds, colours and great possibilities, can change if only they can be given the right level of support. With that support we have already seen great strides forward in the health and well-being, and indeed education, of the people who live there.

But the best is yet to come...

Note

[1] The CDs were part of the Topics in International Health series published by CABI on behalf of Wellcome Trust.

References

Chapter 2

Jordan, P. and Webbe, G. (1993) Epidemiology. In: Jordan, P., Webbe, G. and Sturrock, R. (eds) *Human Schistosomiasis*. CAB International, Wallingford, UK, pp. 87–158.

King, C.H., Dickman, K. and Tisch, D.J. (2005) Reassessment of the cost of chronic helmintic infection: a meta-analysis of disability-related outcomes in endemic schistosomiasis. *The Lancet* 365, 1561–1569.

Kjetland, E.F., Kurewa, E.N., Ndhlovu, P.D., Midzi, N., Gwanzura, L. *et al.* (2008) Female genital schistosomiasis – a differential diagnosis to sexually transmitted disease: genital itch and vaginal discharge as indicators of genital *Schistosoma haematobium* morbidity in a cross-sectional study in endemic rural Zimbabwe. *Tropical Medicine & International Health* 13, 1509–1517.

Koukounari, A., Fenwick, A., Whawell, S., Kabatereine, N.B., Kazibwe, F. *et al.* (2006) Morbidity indicators of *Schistosoma mansoni*: relationship between infection and anemia in Ugandan schoolchildren before and after praziquantel and albendazole chemotherapy. *American Journal of Tropical Medicine and Hygiene* 75, 278–286.

Leiper, R.T. (1915) Report on the results of the bilharzia mission in Egypt, 1915. *Journal of the Royal Army Medical Corps* 25, 1–48.

Madden, F. (1910) The incidence of bilharziosis in Egypt and its clinical manifestation. *British Medical Journal* 2596, 965–969.

Miyairi, K. and Suzuki, M. (1913) On the development of *Schistosoma japonicum. Tokyo Iji Shinshi* [the Tokyo Medical Journal] 1836, 1961–1965.

Nunn, J.F. and Tapp, E. (2000) Meeting at Manson House, London, 21 May 1998. Tropical diseases in ancient Egypt. *Transactions of the Royal Society of Tropical Medicine and Hygiene* 94, 147–153.

Ruffer, M. (1910) Note on the presence of *Bilharzia haematobia* in Egyptian mummies of the twentieth dynasty (1250–1000 BC). *British Medical Journal* 1, 16.

Chapter 3

Fenwick, A. (1969) Baboons as reservoir hosts of *Schistosoma mansoni. Transactions of the Royal Society of Tropical Medicine and Hygiene* 63, 557.

Fenwick, A. (1971) The control of *S. mansoni* on a sugar estate in Tanzania. *East African Medical Journal* 48, 447.

Fenwick, A. (1972a) The costs and cost-benefit analysis of an *S. mansoni* control programme on an irrigated estate in Tanzania. *Bulletin of the World Health Organization* 47, 573–578.

Fenwick, A. (1972b) Effect of control programme on transmission of *S. mansoni* on an irrigated estate in Tanzania. *Bulletin of the World Health Organization* 47, 325–330.

Fenwick, A. and Figenschou, H. (1972) The effect of *S. mansoni* infection on the productivity of cane cutters on a sugar estate in Tanzania. *Bulletin of the World Health Organization* 47, 567.

Fenwick, A. and Jorgennesen, T.A. (1972) The effect of a control programme against *S. mansoni* on the prevelance and intensity of infection on an irrigated estate in Tanzania. *Bulletin of the World Health Organization* 47, 579.

Fenwick, A. and Lidgate, H.J. (1970) Attempts to eradicate snails from impounded water by the use of N-trityl morpholine. *Bulletin of the World Health Organization* 42, 581.

Guzman, M.A., Rugel, A.R., Tarpley, R.S., Alwan, S.N., Chevalier, F.D. *et al.* (2020) An iterative process produces oxamniquine derivatives that kill the major species of schistosomes infecting humans. *PLOS Neglected Tropical Diseases* 14, e0008517.

Chapter 4

Amin, M. and Fenwick, A. (1975) Aerial applications of N-trityl morpholine to irrigation canals in Sudan. *Annals of Tropical Medicine and Parasitology* 69, 257.

Amin, M. and Fenwick, A. (1977) The development of an annual regime for blanket snail control on the Gezira Irrigated Area, in Sudan. *Annals of tropical Medicine and Parasitology* 71, 205–212.

Amin, M.A., Fenwick, A., Osgerby, J.M., Warley, A.P. and Wright, A.N. (1976) A large scale snail control trial with trifenmorph in the Gezira Scheme, Sudan. *Bulletin of the World Health Organization* 54, 573–585.

Chevalier, F.D., Clec'h, W.L., McDew-White, M., Manon, V., Guzman, M.A. *et al.* (2019) Oxamniquine resistance alleles are widespread in Old World *Schistosoma mansoni* and predate drug deployment. *PLOS Pathogens* 15, e1007881.

Christopherson, J.B. (1919) The cure of bilharzia disease by intravenous injections of antimony tartrate: the prophylactic action of the drug. *British Medical Journal* 2, 494.

el Gaddal, A. (1985) The Blue Nile Health Project: a comprehensive approach to the prevention and control of water-associated diseases in irrigated schemes of the Sudan. *Journal of Tropical Medicine and Hygiene* 88, 47–56.

Fenwick, A. and Amin, M. (1982) Marking snails with nail varnish as a field experimental technique. *Annals of Tropical Medicine and Parasitology* 77, 387.

Fenwick, A., Keiser, J. and Utzinger, J. (2006) Epidemiology, burden and control of schistosomiasis with particular consideration to past and current treatment trends. *Drugs of the Future* 31, 413–425.

Fenwick, A., Savioli, L., Engels, D., Bergquist, N.R. and Todd, M.H. (2003) Drugs for the control of parasitic diseases: current status and development in schistosomiasis. *Trends in Parasitology* 19, 509–515.

Kardaman, M.W., Amin, M.A., Fenwick, A., Cheesmond, A.K. and Dixon, H.G. (1983) A field trial using praziquantel (BiltricidieR) to treat *Schistosoma mansoni* and *Schistosoma haematobium* infection in the Gezira, Sudan. *Annals of Tropical Medicine and Parasitology* 77, 297–304.

Omer, A., Hamilton, P., Marshall, T. and Draper, C. (1976) Infection with *Schistosoma mansoni* in the Gezira area of the Sudan. *Journal of Tropical Medicine and Hygiene* 79, 151–157.

Osman, M., Shehab, A., Zaki, A. and Farag, H. (2011) Evaluation of two doses of triclabendazole in treatment of patients with combined schistosomiasis and fascioliasis. *East Mediterranean Health Journal* 17, 266–270.

Chapter 5

El Khoby, T., Galal, N. and Fenwick, A. (1998) The USAID/Government of Egypt's Schistosomiasis Research Project (SRP). *Parasitology Today* 14, 92–96.

Fenwick, A. (2017) Schistosomiasis research and control since the retirement of Sir Patrick Manson in 1914. *Transactions of the Royal Society of Tropical Medicine and Hygiene* 111, 191–198.

Schistosomiasis Research Project (2000) Schistosomiasis in Egypt. *American Journal of Tropical Medicine and Hygiene* 62, 99.

Chapter 7

Coulibaly, J.T., N'Gbesso, Y.K., Knopp, S., N'Guessan, A. and Silué, K.D. *et al.* (2013) Accuracy of urine circulating cathodic antigen test for the diagnosis of *Schistosoma mansoni* in preschool-aged children before and after treatment. *PLOS Neglected Tropical Diseases* 7, e2109.

Montresor, A., Engels, D., Chitsulo, L., Bundu, D.A., Brooker, S. and Savioli, L. (2001) Development and validation of a 'tablet pole' for the administration of praziquantel in sub-Saharan Africa. *Transactions Royal Society of Tropical Medicine and Hygiene* 95, 542–544.

Utzinger, J., Becker, S.L., Van Lieshout, L., Van Dam, G.J. and Knopp, S. (2015) New diagnostic tools in schistosomiasis. *Clinical Microbiology Infection* 6, 529–542.

Chapter 8

Hotez, P.J. (2008) *Forgotten People, Forgotten Diseases: The Neglected Tropical Diseases and Their Impact on Global Health and Development.* American Society of Microbiology, Washington, DC.

Hotez, P., Otteson, A., Fenwick, A. and Molyneux, D. (2006) The neglected tropical diseases: the ancient afflictions of stigma and poverty and the prospects of their control and elimination. *Advances in Experimental Medicine and Biology* 582, 23–33.

Hotez, P., Raff, S., Fenwick, A., Richards, F. and Molyneux, D.H. (2007) Recent progress in integrated neglected tropical disease control. *Trends in Parasitology* 23, 511–514.

Lammie, P., Fenwick, A. and Utzinger, J. (2006) A blueprint for success: integration of neglected tropical disease control programmes. *Trends in Parasitology* 22, 313–321.

Chapter 9

Fenwick, A. (2006) Implementation of human schistosomiasis control: challenges and prospects. *Advances In Parasitology* 61, 576–622.

Montresor, A., Engels, D., Ramsan, M., Foum, A. and Savioli, L. (2002) Field test of the 'dose pole' for praziquantel in Zanzibar. *Transactions of The Royal Society of Tropical Medicine and Hygiene* 96, 323–324.

Van der Werf, M.J., de Vlas, S.J., Landouré, A., Bosopem, K.M. and Habbema, J.D.F. (2004) Measuring schistosomiasis case management of the health services in Ghana and Mali. *Tropical Medicine and International Health* 9, 149–157.

Chapter 10

Bergquist, R. and Whittaker, M. (2012) Control of neglected tropical diseases in Asia Pacific: implications for health information priorities. *Infectious Diseases of Poverty* 1(3).

Gabrielli, A.-F., Touré, S., Sellin, E., Ky, C. Ouedraogo, H. *et al.* (2006) A combined school- and community-based campaign targeting all school-age children of Burkina Faso against schistosomiasis and soil-transmitted helminthiasis: performance, financial costs and implications for sustainability. *Acta Tropica* 99, 234–242.

Garba, A., Touré, S., Dembelé, R., Bosque-Oliva, E. and Fenwick, A. (2006) Implementation of national schistosomiasis control programmes in West Africa. *Trends in Parasitology* 22, 322–326.

Touré, S., Zhang, Y., Bosqué-Oliva, E., Ky, C. and Ouedraogo, A. (2008) Two-year impact of single praziquantel treatment on infection in the national control programme on schistosomiasis in Burkina Faso. *Bulletin of the World Health Organization* 86, 780–787.

Chapter 11

Berhe, N., Gundersen, S.G., Abebe, F., Birrie, H., Medhin, G. and Gemetchu, T. (1999) Praziquantel side effects and efficacy related to Schistosoma mansoni egg loads and morbidity in primary school children in North-East Ethiopia. *Acta Tropica*, 7253–7263.

Cioli, D. and Pica-Mattoccia, L. (2003) Praziquantel. *Parasitology Research* 90, S3–9.

Clements, A.C.A., Lwambo, N.J.S., Blair, L., Nyandindi, U., Kaatano, G. *et al.* (2006) Bayesian spatial analysis and disease mapping: tools to enhance planning and implementation of a schistosomiasis control programme in Tanzania. *Tropical Medicine & International Health* 11, 490–503.

Clements, A.C.A., Garba, A., Sacko, M., Touré, S., Dembelé, R. *et al.* (2008) Mapping the probability of schistosomiasis and associated uncertainty, West Africa. *Emerging Infectious Diseases* 14, 1629–1632.

Frohberg, H. (1984) Results of toxicological studies on praziquantel. *Arzneimittel-Forschung* 34, 1137–1144.

Olds, G.R., King, C., Hewlett, J., Olveda, R., Wu, G. *et al.* (1999) Double-blind placebo-controlled study of concurrent administration of albendazole and praziquantel in schoolchildren with schistosomiasis and geohelminths. *Journal of Infectious Diseases* 179, 996–1003.

Polderman, A.M., Gryseels, B., Gerold, J.L., Mpamila, K. and Manshande, J.P. (1984) Side effects of praziquantel in the treatment of *Schistosoma mansoni* in Maniema, Zaire. *Transactions of the Royal Society of Tropical Medicine and Hygiene* 78, 752–754.

Webbe, G. (1962) The transmission of *Schistosoma haematobium* in an area of Lake Province, Tanganyika. *Bulletin of the World Health Organization* 27, 59–85.

Chapter 12

Morgan, S., Bathula, H.S. and Moon, S. (2020) Pricing of pharmaceuticals is becoming a major challenge for health systems. *British Medical Journal* 368, l4627.

Chapter 14

Ahuja, A., Baird, S., Hamory Hicks, J. and Miguel, E. (2017) Economics of mass deworming programmes. In: Bundy, D.A.P., de Silva, N., Horton, S., Jamison, D.T. and Patton, G. (eds) *Disease Control Priorities*, 3rd edn. World Bank, Washington, DC.

Brooker, S., Kabatereine, N.B., Fleming, F. and Devlin, N. (2008) Cost and cost-effectiveness of nationwide school-based helminth control in Uganda: intra-country variation and effects of scaling-up. *Health Policy and Planning* 23, 24–35.

Hotez, P.J. (2008) *Forgotten People, Forgotten Diseases: The Neglected Tropical Diseases and Their Impact on Global Health and Development*. American Society of Microbiology, Washington, DC.

Kabatereine, N.B., Brooker, S., Koukounari, A., Kazibwe, F., Tukahebwa, E. *et al.* (2007) Impact of a national helminth control programme on infection and morbidity in Ugandan schoolchildren. *Bulletin of the World Health Organisation* 85, 91–99.

Koukounari, A., Gabrielli, A.F., Touré, S., Bosque-Oliva, E., Zhang, Y. *et al.* (2007) *Schistosoma haematobium* infection and morbidity before and after large-scale administration of praziquantel in Burkina Faso. *Journal of Infectious Diseases* 196, 659–669.

Nokes, C., Grantham-McGregor, S.M., Sawyer, A.W., Cooper, E.S. and Bundy, D.A. (1992) Parasitic helminth infection and cognitive function in schoolchildren. *Proceedings: Biological Sciences* 247, 77–81.

Sakti, H., Nokes, C., Hertanto, W.S., Hendranto, S., Hall, A., Bundy, D.A and Satoto (1999) Evidence for an association between hookworm infection and cognitive function in Indonesian schoolchildren. *Tropical Medicine and International Health* 4, 322–334.

Seward, N. (2007) *Mali Three-year Data Internal Report to SCI*, s.l.: s.n.

Stephenson, L. (1993) The impact of schistosomiasis on human nutrition. *Parasitology* 107, S107–S123.

Vennervald, B.J. and Dunne, D.W. (2004) Morbidity in schistosomiasis: an update. *Current Opinions in Infectious Disease* 17, 439–447.

Zhang, Y., Koukounari, A., Kabatereine, N., Fleming, F., Kazibwe, F. *et al.* (2007) Parasitological impact of two-year preventive chemotherapy on schistosomiasis and soil-transmitted helminthiasis in Uganda. *BMC Medicine* 5, 27.

Chapter 16

Adriko, M. (2014) Evaluation of circulating cathodic antigen (CCA) urine-cassette assay as a survey tool for *Schistosoma mansoni* in different transmission settings within Bugiri District, Uganda. *Acta Tropica* 136, 50–57.

Engels, D., Chitsulo, L., Montresor, A. and Savioli, L. (2002) The global epidemiological situation of schistosomiasis and new approaches to control and research. *Acta Tropica* 82, 139–146.

Chapter 17

Brown, P. (1994) Deadly worm may be turning drug-resistant. *New Scientist* 144, 4.

Colley, D.G. and Secor, W.E. (2007) A schistosomiasis research agenda. *PLOS Neglected Tropical Diseases* 1, e32.

Colley, D.G., Jacobson, J.A. and Binder, S. (2020) Schistosomiasis Consortium for Operational Research and Evaluation (SCORE): its foundations, development, and evolution. *American Journal of Tropical Medicine and Hygiene* 103, 5–13.

Danso-Appiah, A. and De Vlas, S.J. (2002) Interpreting low praziquantel cure rates of *Schistosoma mansoni* infections in Senegal. *Trends in Parasitology* 18, 125–129.

Davies, C.M., Fairbrother, E. and Webster, J.P. (2002) Mixed strain schistosome infections of snails and the evolution of parasite virulence. *Parasitology* 124, 31–38.

Doenhoff, M.J. and Pica-Mattoccia, L. (2006) Praziquantel for the treatment of schistosomiasis: its use for control in areas with endemic disease and prospects for drug resistance. *Expert Review of Anti-infective Therapy* 4, 199–210.

Fallon, P.G. and Doenhoff, M.J. (1994) Drug-resistant schistosomiasis: resistance to praziquantel and oxamniquine induced in *Schistosoma mansoni* in mice is drug specific. *American Journal of Tropical Medicine and Hygiene* 51, 83–88.

Gower, C.M. and Webster, J.P. (2005) Intraspecific competition and the evolution of virulence in a parasitic trematode. *Evolution. International Journal of Organic Evolution* 59, 544–553.

Gryseels, B., Mbaye, A., de Vlas, S.J., Stelma, F.F., Guissé, F. et al. (2001) Are poor responses to praziquantel for the treatment of *Schistosoma mansoni* infections in Senegal due to resistance? An overview of the evidence. *Tropical Medicine and International Health* 6, 864–873.

Ismail, M., Botros, S., Metwally, A., Williams, S., Farghally, A. et al. (1999) Resistance to praziquantel: direct evidence from *Schistosoma mansoni* isolated from Egyptian villagers. *American Journal of Tropical Medicine and Hygiene* 60, 932–935.

Ismail, M., Metwally, A., Farghally, A., Bruce, J., Tao, L.F., and Bennett, J.L. (1996) Characterization of isolates of *Schistosoma mansoni* from Egyptian villagers that tolerate high doses of praziquantel. *American Journal of Tropical Medicine and Hygiene* 55, 214–218.

Kabatereine, N.B., Brooker, S., Koukounari, A., Kazibwe, F., Tukahebwa, E. et al. (2007) Impact of a national helminth control programme on infection and morbidity in Ugandan schoolchildren. *Bulletin of the World Health Organization* 85, 91–99.

Mutapi, F., Ndhlovu, P.D., Hagan, P. and Woolhouse, M.E. (1998) Changes in specific anti-egg antibody levels following treatment with praziquantel for *Schistosoma haematobium* infection in children. *Parasite Immunology* 20, 595–600.

Ribeiro dos Santos, G., Verjovski-Almeida, S. and Leite, L.C.C. (2006) Schistosomiasis: a century searching for chemotherapeutic drugs. *Parasitology Research* 99, 505–521.

Webster, J.P. and Davies, C.M. (2001) Coevolution and compatibility in the snail-schistosome system. *Parasitology* 123, S41–56.

Webster, J.P., Shrivastava, J., Johnson, P.J. and Blair, L. (2007) Is host-schistosome coevolution going anywhere? *BMC Evolutionary Biology* 7, 91.

Woolhouse, M.E.J., Webster, J.P., Domingo, E., Charlesworth, B. and Levin, B.R. (2002) Biological and biomedical implications of the co-evolution of pathogens and their hosts. *Nature Genetics* 32, 569–577.

Chapter 19

Babu, S. and Nutman, T. (2016) Helminth-tuberculosis co-infection: an immunologic perspective. *Trends in Immunology* 37, 597–607.

Baker, M.C., Mathieu, E., Fleming, F.M., Deming, M., King, J.D. et al. (2010) Mapping, monitoring, and surveillance of neglected tropical diseases: towards a policy framework. *The Lancet* 375, 231–238.

Brooker, S., Clements, A.C.A., Hotez, P., Hay, S., Tatem, A. *et al.* (2006) The co-distribution of *Plasmodium falciparum* and hookworm among African schoolchildren. *Malaria Journal* 5, 99.

Cadmus, S.I., Akinseye, V.O., Taiwo, B.O., Pinelli, E.O., Van Soolingen, D. and Rhodes, S. (2020) Interactions between helminths and tuberculosis infections: implications for tuberculosis diagnosis and vaccination in Africa. *PLOS Neglected Tropical Diseases* 14, e0008069.

Druilhe, P., Tall, A. and Sokhna, C. (2005) Worms can worsen malaria: towards a new means to roll back malaria? *Trends in Parasitology* 21, 359–362.

Fenwick, A., Molyneux, D. and Nantulya, V. (2005) Achieving the millennium development goals. *The Lancet* 365, 1029–1030.

Fincham, J.E., Markus, M. and Adams, V.J. (2003) Could control of soil-transmitted helminthic infection influence the HIV/AIDS pandemic. *Acta Tropica* 86, 315–333.

Fitzpatrick, C., Fleming, F.M., Madin-Warburton, M., Schneider, T., Meheus, F. *et al.* (2016) Benchmarking the cost per person of mass treatment for selected neglected tropical diseases: an approach based on literature review and meta-regression with web-based software application. *PLOS Neglected Tropical Diseases* 10, e0005037.

Harding-Esch, E., Brady, M.A., Angeles, C.A.C., Fleming, F.M., Martin, D.L. *et al.* (2021) Lessons from the field: integrated survey methodologies for neglected tropical diseases. *Transactions of the Royal Society for Tropical Medicine and Hygiene* 115, 124–126.

Hotez, P.J., Molyneux, D.H., Fenwick, A., Ottesen, E., Ehrlich, S. and Sachs, J.D. (2006) Incorporating a rapid-impact package for neglected tropical diseases with programs for HIV/AIDS, tuberculosis, and malaria. *PLOS Medicine* 3, e102.

Hotez, P.J., Fenwick, A. and Molyneux, D.H. (2021) The new COVID-19 poor and the neglected tropical diseases resurgence. *Infectious Diseases of Poverty* 10, 10.

Kabatereine, N.B., Malecela, M., Lado, M., Zarmaba, S., Amiel, O. and Kolaczinski, J.H. (2010) How to (or not to) integrate vertical programmes for the control of major neglected tropical diseases in sub-Saharan Africa. *PLOS Neglected Tropical Diseases* 4, e755.

Maizels, R. and McSorley, H. (2016) Regulation of the host immune system by helminth parasites. *Journal of Allergy and Clinical Immunology* 138, 666–675.

Molyneux, D.H., Hotez, P.J. and Fenwick, A. (2005) 'Rapid-impact interventions': how a policy of integrated control for Africa's neglected tropical diseases could benefit the poor. *PLOS Medicine* 2, e336.

Molyneux, D.H., Aboe, A., Isiyaku, S. and Bush, S. (2020) COVID-19 and neglected tropical diseases in Africa: impacts, interactions, consequences. *International Health* 12, 367–372.

WHO (2015) Investing to overcome the global impact of neglected tropical diseases.

Zakeri, A., Hansen, E.P., Andersen, S.D., Williams, A.R. and Nejsum, P. (2018) Immunomodulation by helminths: intracellular pathways and extracellular vesicles. *Frontiers in Immunology* 9, 2349. DOI: 10.3389/fimmu.2018.02349.

Chapter 20

Global Schistosomiasis Alliance (2021) The Pediatric Praziquantel Consortium receives funding for the ADOPT programme, for the treatment of schistosomiasis in preschool-aged children. [Online]. Available at: www.eliminateschisto.org/news-events/news/ped iatric-praziquantel-consortium-funding-adopt-programme (accessed 1 September 2021).

Index

Page numbers in *italics* refer to illustrations. AF = Alan Fenwick.